PHYSIOTHERAPY IN COMMON UPPER EXTREMITY CONDITIONS

EVIDENCE BASED APPROACH

NIHAR RANJAN MOHANTY

Copyright © NIHAR RANJAN MOHANTY
All Rights Reserved.

ISBN 978-1-64783-463-0

This book has been published with all efforts taken to make the material error-free after the consent of the author. However, the author and the publisher do not assume and hereby disclaim any liability to any party for any loss, damage, or disruption caused by errors or omissions, whether such errors or omissions result from negligence, accident, or any other cause.

While every effort has been made to avoid any mistake or omission, this publication is being sold on the condition and understanding that neither the author nor the publishers or printers would be liable in any manner to any person by reason of any mistake or omission in this publication or for any action taken or omitted to be taken or advice rendered or accepted on the basis of this work. For any defect in printing or binding the publishers will be liable only to replace the defective copy by another copy of this work then available.

DEDICATED TO MY BELOVED PARENTS

Nihar Ranjan Mohanty

BPT; [Swami Vivekanand National Institute Of Rehabilitation Training And Research, Cuttack, Odisha, India]

MPT (Sports); [Guru Nanak Dev University, Amritsar, Punjab, India]

Contents

Preface — vii
Acknowledgements — ix

1. Lateral Epicondylitis — 1
2. Medial Elbow Pain — 10
3. Olecranon Bursitis — 23
4. Rotator-cuff Injury — 44
5. Cubital Tunnel Syndrome — 54
6. Carpal Tunnel Syndrome — 61
7. Rotator Cuff Calcific Tendinitis — 69
8. Physiotherapy In Cubital Tunnel Syndrome — 76
9. Physiotherapy In Frozen Shoulder — 80
10. Focal Task Specific Dystonia — 85
11. Bibliography — 92

Preface

This Book is a clear approach towards evidence based practice of upper extremity conditions. Most common upper extremiity problems are discussed with recent evidences. The language is lucid and written in a very concise manner. Point-wise presentation of the subject matters is the strength of this book. Physiotherapist can use this book as a handy material for all the common problems of upper extremities.

Acknowledgements

First and foremost I would like to thank the almighty for his support and blessings in this long journey.

I would like to express my deepest sense of gratitude to my respected teacher & guide, **Prof. (Dr.) Shyamal Koley**, Head, Department of Physiotherapy, Guru Nanak Dev University, Amritsar, whose knowledge, guidance, and constant encouragement and deep insight without which this book would not have found its final shape.

I would like to thank my **Mother**, for all her support, guidance, motivation and unconditional love, without which I would have never made it through my book. Along with her my greatest regards goes to my **Father, my sisters and my brothers** for the confidence they had in me and I am at loss of words to convey my appreciation and warm regards to them.

My sincere thanks go to my friends **Avinash Tiwari** for helping me in my book and being with me in need.

Nihar Ranjan Mohanty

CHAPTER ONE

LATERAL EPICONDYLITIS

INTRODUCTION

Lateral epicondylopathy, or tennis elbow is a common cause of lateral elbow pain in the general population and in athletes, with a reported prevalence as high as 3.5 per 1000 people. The condition occurs classically with degeneration of the extensor carpi radialis brevis (ECRB) origin on the lateral epicondyle. Extensor tendons, including the supinator, extensor carpi radialis longus, and the extensor digitorum can also be involved.

It is thought that the condition results from chronic overuse and is often seen in tennis players, heavy labourers, and even string musicians. Tennis in particular can place strain on the elbow through the high forces and torque experienced while striking the ball with the player's racket. It has also been reported that up to 50% of all tennis players may experience this condition. It is more common in older, professional athletes than amateur athletes but it can be seen at all ages.

Multiple theories exist as to the cause of lateral epicondylopathy. Primarily it is considered a condition of overuse; however in tennis it may be due to the force of striking the ball that hits the racket causing the forearm muscles to experience eccentric loading and micro trauma. The distinct tennis backhand also contributes largely to the lateral sided loading. This may be more pronounced in amateur players as it has been found that they are more likely to hit a backhand using a flexed wrist versus more experienced players.

Although previously believed to be an inflammatory process within the forearm extensor tendons, it has been shown that within the pathologic tendons there is a lack of inflammatory cells. Histologically, tendons involved show disorganized collagen structure, fibroblast hypertrophy and vascular hyperplasia. The pathologic tissue is usually on the deeper surfaces of the tendon closer to the centre of force or rotation relative to the muscle load and joint movement.

AETIOLOGY AND PATHOGENESIS

In the majority of cases, non-obvious underlying causes can be identified. Extensor carpi radialis brevis (ECRB) is the most commonly affected muscle, but supinator and other wrist extensors such as extensor carpi radialis longus, extensor digitorum, extensor digiti minimi and extensor carpi ulnaris can be involved. Any activity involving excessive and repetitive use of these muscles (for example tennis, playing an instrument, typing, manual work) may cause the tendinosis. Smoking and obesity have been identified as significant risk factors. Though LE was classically identified as an inflammatory process, the histology does not show many inflammatory cells; most authors therefore consider LE as a tendinosis, a symptomatic degenerative process of the tendon. The application of tension to a tendon usually increases cross-linkage and collagen deposition. Tendons can stretch easily in response to gradually increasing forces. If this stress exceeds the tendon's tolerance to stretch, a microtear may occur. Multiple microtears lead to degenerative changes within the tendon which are known as tendinosis. Histological changes such as angiofibroblastic hyperplasia (a manifestation of granulation tissue that disturbs correct collagen synthesis) can also be seen. Histopathological studies of ECRB in patients with long-standing LE have shown necrosis as well as signs of fibre regeneration. Nevertheless, additional pathophysiological mechanisms have been suggested.

Painful symptomatic LE can result in underuse of the tendon. Underuse changes the tendon structure, leading to progressive weakening and increasing the risk of injury. In conjunction with underuse, shearing forces lead to fibrocartilaginous formation at the ECRB enthesis, which contributes to weakening at the tendon-bone junction. In addition, the tendon vascularisation is deficient and sustained muscle contractions can lead to tendon ischaemia. Repetitive activities increase temperature which can lead to hyperthermic injuries of the enthesis. Despite all of these considerations, there is a lack of knowledge to explain the great variability of symptoms among patients. Peripheral nerve irritation and local altered pain response have been proposed. Shoulder and neck pain are frequent symptoms in this population, but they can be associated with alterations in upper limb biomechanics.

CLINICAL PRESENTATION

Lateral epicondylopathy is one of the most common causes of lateral elbow pain in patients. The patient often presents with pain on resisted extension, such as hitting a backhand shot, lifting heavy objects, or when is using a screwdriver. They may also complain of pain with strong grip, or even with decreased grip strength. Workers and labourers may complain of pain with duties that require repetitive wrist extension. Range of motion is often preserved and no gross deformities are usually seen with inspection.

It is important to differentiate lateral epicondylopathy from other conditions that may affect the elbow. Cervical radiculopathy may cause radiating pain to the elbow. Radial tunnel syndrome may also be a concurrent finding with lateral epicondylopathy and must be properly differentiated. Key findings for radial tunnel syndrome are pain more distal to the forearm extensor mass orgin (greater than 3 cm) compared to lateral epicondylopathy, as well as paresthesias or pain in the hand.

Clinical conditions that mimic lateral epicondylopathy include degenerative joint disease, osteochondritis dissecans, elbow overuse, lateral and posterolateral elbow instability, and even anconeus inflammation. When pain is refractory to conservative approaches, a broader differential diagnosis must be entertained. There appears to be a high incidence of refractory lateral elbow pain (up to 59%) with patients with underlying osteochondral defects.

A number of provocative tests can be employed during physical examination, on top of palpation at the lateral epicondyle. These include Maudsley's test and Cozen's maneuver, with sensitivities of 66% and 91% respectively. Maudsley's test involves having the patient perform resisted extension of the long finger while the examiner palpates the lateral condyle. A positive test recreates the pain. Cozen's maneuver is similar and is positive when pain is elicited with resisted wrist extension while the elbow is extended to isolate the ECRB.

IMAGING

The diagnosis of lateral epicondylopathy is a clinical one. Given the history, physical exam, and positive provocative tests the diagnosis can be made. If there is concern for a congruent or separate etiology more diagnostic imaging can be undertaken. Radiographs are often normal, and may be employed if there is concern for bony abnormalities such as loose bodies or osteochondral defects (OCD).

Ultrasound is also useful to rule out the disease. Often times if no tendon changes including neovascularization, thinning, thickening or tears are identified on ultrasound then an alternate diagnosis should be sought. Sensitivity of ultrasound imaging ranges from 64-82% and specificity ranges from 67-100%.

Magnetic resonance imaging (MRI) is often used to better clarify anatomic pathology including edema in the ERCB tendon, tendonopathic changes, underlying OCD lesions, or edema in the insertion onto the epicondyle. Sensitivity in MRI is greater than ultrasound at 90- 100% while specificity is similar at 83-100%. The clinician needs to interpret MRI findings with caution as clinical symptoms and MRI findings may not always be congruent in their severity.

DIFERENTIAL DIAGNOSIS

In a middle-aged patient with pain on the lateral side of the elbow and typical symptoms and signs, lateral epicondylitis should undoubtedly be the main diagnosis, but one must rule out other potential conditions which can cause lateral pain. The following should be considered:

1. Cervical radiculopathy with pain in the elbow and forearm.

2. Elbow overuse to compensate for a disease in an adjacent joint (frozen shoulder for example).

3. Posterior interosseous nerve (PIN) entrapment (also known as 'radial tunnel syndrome'). Nerve compression produces neuropathic pain in the lateral forearm. However, pain is not reproduced by wrist extension. Resisted supination can produce pain as the supinator is one of the possible areas of PIN compression. An anaesthetic block of PIN can be diagnostic, but injection should be performed selectively to avoid diffusion of the local anaesthetic to the lateral epicondyle area. The middle finger extension test, resisted supination of the forearm and nerve conduction studies have all been described to assist in the diagnosis of radial tunnel syndrome.

4. Degenerative changes and OCD of the capitellum. It has been observed that 59% of cases of lateral elbow pain refractory to conservative treatment have some chondral changes in the radiocapitellar joint. OCD typically affects young individuals involved in sports and physical activities who have mild grinding and pain when performing a moving valgus test.

5. Inflammation and oedema of the anconeus muscle. Some studies have reported a relatively high incidence of anconeus oedema, shown in MRI of patients complaining of lateral elbow pain. Fasciotomy of the muscle can solve that problem.

6. Posterolateral elbow instability should definitely be ruled out in every patient suffering from lateral elbow pain. The association between

instability and epicondylitis has been established, following excessive use of steroids or the local pathogenic insult. The presentation is low-grade and may require examination of the patient under anesthesia to test it properly. The presence of cubitus varus, previous surgery or dislocations of the elbow should be assessed.

7. Other causes of pain include low-grade infection (*Propionibacterium acnes*) or other inflammatory diseases such as rheumatoid arthritis.

NON-OPERATIVE TREATMENT

There are multiple treatment modalities for lateral epicondylopathy. A very high success rate can be expected with classic non-operative treatment, which includes the following physical and rehabilitation modalities:

1. *Activity Modification, Rest, Ice*

These modalities are the initial treatment of any case of lateral epicondylopathy. The athlete should reduce their load intensity when symptoms present with early treatments targeted initial injury and appropriate time to healing. Loading assessment including frequency and intensity should be carefully monitored and controlled on the athlete's return to play. Modifications to the way the patient plays the game of tennis can include things such as two fisted compared to a single fisted backhand, a more flexible or shock absorbent racquet designs, lower string tension, selecting a slower playing court surface, broader racquets with larger sweet spots, as well as modifying the racquet to larger grips have all been done to target a decreased strain on the extensor muscle mass.

2. *Physiotherapy* is another alternative. There are various modalities via physical therapy treatment for tennis elbow. As is the case for most tendinopathies, eccentric strengthening should be among the cornerstones of treatment, with adjuvant stretching of the extensor mass also shown to be helpful. Strengthening and optimizing all links of the kinetic chain (core, shoulder, and scapula) is fundamental to the treatment of most elbow injuries since the kinetic chain so often contributes to the problem.

Deep friction massage, electrical stimulation, cryotherapy and dry needling are alternative treatments that can be provided by the therapist who is trying to target the underlying process and motivate a healing response.

Dry needling has shown short term benefits (2-8weeks) but no long term differences versus placebo. There have been limited long-term studies for manipulation and stretching of the extensor mass; however in the short term it does appear to be helpful in reducing pain.

Eccentric exercises and partial load-favouring tendon healing are the mainstay of physiotherapy regimes. A stable shoulder and scapula are necessary for correct elbow function; strengthening exercises of the scapular stabilisers including the lower trapezius, serratus anterior and rotator cuff muscles is mandatory.

3. *Epicondylar counterforce braces* work by reducing tension in the wrist extensors. Elbow straps, clasps or sleeve orthoses have been demonstrated as superior for pain relief and grip strength when compared with placebo orthoses.[27] However, no differences between braces were shown in a systematic review[28] and we do not use them in our practice. We have seen patients with secondary nerve problems due to prolonged use of a counterforce brace.

4. *Non-steroidal anti-inflammatory drugs* (NSAIDs) can be useful for the short-term relief of symptoms. Even if their use is superior to a placebo, no differences between oral and topical NSAIDs have been established.[29]

5. *Corticosteroid injections* are commonly used to treat LE. The way in which they work is currently unknown; they probably help to control local inflammatory response and pain mediation.[30] Corticosteroid injections seem to be superior to NSAIDs at four weeks, but no differences are observed at a later stage. Cortisone injections should be avoided in all cases, unless a short-term good result is advisable (such as a professional tennis player in mid-season), as most patients improve without corticosteroids and better long-term results can be achieved without them.[31] Patients should be advised of potential side-effects including changes in colouration of the skin, fat atrophy and muscle wasting.

6. *Autologous blood injections* are thought to work by stimulating an inflammatory response which will bring in the necessary nutrients to promote healing. Short-term good results have been reported recently;[32,33] however, no benefit in the long-term follow-up has been found and its use is only recommended for those recalcitrant cases when other modalities of treatment have failed.

7. *Platelet-rich plasma injections* (PRP). These preparations are thought to contain high concentrations of growth factors, which could theoretically enhance tendon healing. General technique involves patient blood extraction, centrifugation and re-injection of the plasma into the lateral epicondyle. Good outcomes have been reported.[34,35] However, no differences were seen between PRP and whole blood injections.[36]

Moreover, significant differences among available commercial systems and variations in the technique make it difficult to draw clear conclusions about the use of PRP in this pathology. New legal regulations could slow down the adoption of these last techniques.

8. *Percutaneous radiofrequency thermal treatment*. A radiofrequency electrode is introduced percutaneously under ultrasound guidance which produces a thermal injury when activated, inducing a microtenotomy and removing all pathological tissue. Good outcomes have been reported, and no reduction of tendon size has been observed.37

9. *Extracorporeal shock-wave therapy* (ECSW) has been proposed as an alternative to non-operative management. The mechanism of action is not fully known. A generator of specific frequency sound waves is applied directly onto the overlying skin of the ECRB tendon. It has not been demonstrated to be more beneficial than other treatment modalities.

10. *The use of low-level laser therapy* has been proposed due to the stimulating effect of laser on collagen production in tendons. Although laser was not initially viewed as particularly useful among LE therapies, a recent study has demonstrated some short-term benefits when using an adequate dose and wavelength.

11. *Acupuncture* has demonstrated good outcomes on short-term follow-up. However, long-term results remain unclear.

12. *Botulinum toxin A injections* act by diminishing muscle tone. Reducing the tension on the ECRB insertion could be beneficial for pain relief. Good short-term results have been published, but as yet there is no consensus on its use and the effects may be conditioned by the technique, the operator and the dose.

OPERATIVE TREATMENT

Should conservative non-operative treatment fail over a span of six to twelve months, and the symptoms of lateral epicondylitis are debilitating enough for the patient, operative treatment can be undertaken. Although there is no consensus as to the best operative approach (open, arthroscopic or percutaneous), there have been a number of techniques described for treatment.

Open

Multiple open techniques to addressing lateral epicondylopathy have been described. One technique is to expose the ECRB, excise any angio-fibrotic tissue and finally repair the lesion if necessary. Gunn et al. reports a success rate of 85% when defined as return to sport.

Other techniques described include extensor releases, V-Y tendon slide of the ECRB and anconeus excision. No matter the open technique chosen, a lateral approach to the elbow is used, ECRB is identified and debridement, release or a combination of the two with or without repair of the tendon is completed. Denervation of the lateral epicondyle can also be undertaken, with up to 80% success rate, which involves resection of the posterior branches of the posterior cutaneous nerve of the forearm.

Long term analysis of the open release of the extensor tendon over a span of 10 years through a retrospective review has shown positive results. 97% of the 139 procedures completed had improved outcomes postoperatively up to 10 years after the initial procedure in terms of decreased pain, function, and elbow range of motion. The major risk in using the open technique is that extensive release can affect elbow stability if lateral ligaments are attenuated. However, this risk is low, and given the beneficial long term outcomes open surgical release is a useful treatment method should conservative measures fail.

Percutaneous

Percutaneous release offers the benefit of being able to complete the procedure in a quick manner with minimal anesthesia. The technique involves releasing the common extensor mass from the lateral epicondyle. A major disadvantage of this procedure however is that repair is not possible and may limit extension strength. Good outcomes in pain reduction have been reported with this technique however. Although not significant, a systemic review by Pierce et al. found that there may be a better functional outcome with arthroscopic and open release rather than percutaneous approach to lateral epicondylopathy treatment. The review analyzed 848 open, 578 arthroscopic, and 178 percutaneous releases. Scores for the disabilities of the arm, shoulder, and hand were significantly better for open or arthroscopic versus percutaneous. There was also reported to be lower pain scores with percutaneous and arthroscopic than open approach post operatively.

Although the pain scores may initially be lower for the percutaneous approach, it does appear that functional outcomes are not as superior as the other surgical methods. This may be due to the fact that using the percutaneous approach the tendon cannot be repaired after release. Given the high quality systemic review, with over 1,000 cases reported on, it would appear to be more beneficial to undertake an arthroscopic or open surgical procedure for lateral epicondylopathy.

Arthroscopic

Arthroscopic treatment of lateral epicondylopathy is another useful surgical approach. A major advantage of using arthroscopic technique is that the joint can be visualized. If there are intra articular lesions such as loose bodies these can be addressed at the same time as extensor tendon debridement. The viewing portal is placed medially, and the working portal is superolateral.

Szabo et al. showed in a retrospective review that there was no statistical difference between arthroscopic and open treatment of lateral epicondylopathy for pain and functional scores post operatively at a mean follow up of 47.8 months with improvement in Andrews-Carson scores from 160 preoperatively to 195 postoperatively.

With operative treatment there is the possibility of injury to the structures around the elbow. Given the anatomic position of the radial nerve in relation to the operative field, it can be damaged during the procedure. The lateral ulnar collateral ligament can also be damaged, leading to posterolateral instability of the elbow. Therefore debridement should not extend beyond the midline of the radial head to avoid excessive resection of the ligament.

CONCLUSION

Lateral epicondylopathy is one of the most common causes of lateral elbow pain. ECRB irritation and angiofibroblastic changes in the tendon are most commonly attributed to the causation of pain in patients. The mainstay and initial treatment should be non-operative, using rest, bracing and physical therapy, with as high as 90% success rate. When conservative treatment fails, operative treatment can be considered using open or arthroscopic approaches with expected 85-95% success, and better functional outcomes than the percutaneous technique.

CHAPTER TWO

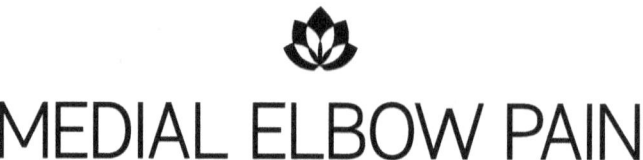

MEDIAL ELBOW PAIN

INTRODUCTION

With the steady increase in the number of participants in overhead-throwing sports over the last few decades, there has been a proportional increase in the incidence of upper extremity injuries among this population. Historically, discussion of overhead-throwing injuries sustained to the elbow has focused on athletes participating in baseball. This has lead to a commonly accepted general term, pitcher's elbow, to describe injuries sustained to the elbow in the throwing athlete. Despite the connotation associated with this nonspecific term, pitcher's elbow can affect any athlete participating in overhead-throwing sports (i.e., softball, football, tennis, javelin, etc.). Due to the complexity of the functional anatomy of the elbow and the significant biomechanical forces generated during a typical throwing cycle, treating clinicians must have a working knowledge of both these topics in order to effectively treat this growing population.

RELEVANT ANATOMY

Stability of the elbow is provided by both bony articulations and soft tissue restraints. The ulno-humeral joint, namely the articulation between the olecranon and the olecranon fossa, is the primary stabilizer at the extremes of elbow motion—flexion less than 20° and greater than 120°. Soft tissue restraints have been shown to provide the primary static and dynamic stability needed in the mid arc of elbow motion. The ulnar collateral ligament (UCL) is the main, soft tissue constraint to valgus instability of the elbow. It is composed of three bundles: anterior bundle, posterior bundle, and transverse bundle. The anterior bundle has been shown to be the primary valgus stabilizer of the UCL between 30° and 120° of flexion, which is when the medial elbow experiences the highest level of valgus force during overhead throwing. The anterior bundle of the UCL is attached proximally at the medial epicondyle of the humerus and attached distally on the sublime tubercle of the proximal ulna. It is subdivided into an anterior band and a posterior band. The anterior band is the primary restraint to valgus stress up to 90° of flexion, while the posterior band becomes increasingly more important as a stabilizer with flexion beyond 90°. The common flexor musculature is comprised of the pronator teres, flexor carpi radialis, palmaris longus, flexor carpi ulnaris, and flexor digitorum superficialis. These muscles originate from the medial epicondyle and act as dynamic stabilizers to valgus forces at the elbow. The ulnar nerve is another medial structure of the elbow that is susceptible to injury in this patient population. The nerve passes the elbow joint within the cubital tunnel, just posterior to the medial epicondyle of the humerus and immediately superficial to the UCL. Ulnar nerve inflammation, compression, or subluxation can lead to severe ulnar nerve symptoms in these athletes that present with pain, numbness, and weakness distally. Lateral stability of the elbow is provided by the radiocapitellar joint, radial collateral ligament, and common extensor muscles. Although lateral-sided injuries in the overhead-throwing athlete are much less common, an understanding of the static and dynamic lateral stabilizers is needed when evaluating these patients.

THROWING BIOMECHANICS

The baseball pitch has been widely studied and can be divided into five main stages. Phase I (windup) involves initial preparation as the elbow flexes and the forearm is slightly pronated. Phase II (early cocking) begins when the ball leaves the glove hand and is complete when the forward foot contacts the ground. Shoulder abduction and external rotation are initiated in this stage. Phase III (late cocking) is characterized by further shoulder abduction and maximal external rotation. Additionally, the elbow flexes between 90° and 120° and the forearm pronates to 90°. Phase IV (rapid acceleration) generates a large forward directed force on the extremity that is accompanied by rapid elbow extension. This stage terminates with ball release. Tremendous valgus stress is generated over the medial aspect of the elbow during this stage, a majority of which is transmitted to the anterior bundle of the UCL. The remainder of the stress is dissipated by the secondary supporting structures of the medial elbow, mainly the flexor-pronator musculature. Phase V (follow-through) involves dissipation of all excess kinetic energy as the elbow reaches full extension and finalizes at completion of motion. Multiple biomechanical studies have shown that the elbow extends over 2300°/s during the throwing cycle. This generates a medial shear force of approximately 300 N and a lateral compressive force of nearly 900 N. Furthermore, in the acceleration phase of the throwing cycle, an additional 64 N of valgus stress is applied to the elbow. These extraordinary forces generated on the elbow joint by the overhead athlete leaves the elbow especially vulnerable to injury. The typical pattern of injury sustained is either due to repetitive microtrauma or chronic stress overload.

VALGUS INSTABILITY

Valgus instability caused by ulnar collateral ligament deficiency is rapidly increasing in incidence. This is easily demonstrated by observing the significant increase in the number of Major League Baseball pitchers who have undergone UCL reconstruction between the years 1986 and 2012. Further proof of this upsurge is noted when considering the alarming increase in high school athletes undergoing this same surgery. Repetitive microtrauma and chronic stress on the medial elbow during the acceleration phase of throwing can lead to laxity and injury to the UCL over time. The anterior bundle of the UCL, as the primary valgus stabilizer of the elbow from 30° to 120°, is most susceptible to injury in these athletes. More specifically, the posterior band of the anterior bundle is taut when the elbow is flexed from 90° to 120°. Since the largest force is generated through the elbow during the acceleration phase (phase IV) when the elbow is flexed from 90° to 100°, the posterior band of the anterior bundle is most commonly effected. Disruption of the UCL can lead to pain, loss of throwing velocity, lack of throwing endurance, and less commonly a subjective sense of instability.

EVALUATION

A thorough history and physical examination are the most important components of the evaluation and diagnosis of an ulnar collateral ligament injury. Radiographic studies are required to confirm this suspected injury. The athlete with an acute UCL injury typically describes the sudden onset of pain with throwing. In approximately 50 % of cases, the patient will report hearing or feeling a pop and are typically unable to continue throwing. More chronic injuries may not present as obvious. They will likely be described as a gradual onset of pain localized to the medial elbow that worsens in the late cocking or early acceleration phase of throwing. A decrease in maximum velocity is also typically reported in chronic cases. Local inflammation of the unstable ligamentous complex can lead to other common elbow complaints such as ulnar nerve symptoms secondary to irritation of the nerve within the cubital tunnel, flexor-pronator mass strain, or medial epicondylitis.

Physical examination should begin with a thorough evaluation of the upper extremity. Proximally, the shoulder should be examined for any deficits in range of motion or rotator cuff symptoms. Additionally, scapular motion and position should be assessed to rule out possible dyskinesia. Examination of the elbow with suspected valgus instability may be performed with the patient seated and the elbow flexed 20–30°. This unlocks the olecranon from its fossa and allows isolated testing of the anterior bundle of the UCL. Palpation is first performed along the UCL as it courses from the medial epicondyle toward the proximal ulna. A slight valgus load is then applied to the elbow and any medial joint space opening may signify potential valgus laxity. If suspected, comparison with the contralateral elbow should be performed. Loss of a firm endpoint that is associated with increased medial joint space opening is consisted with an injured UCL. However, it should be noted thatmost throwing athletes will have a certain degree of increased laxity of the dominant throwing elbow with applied valgus stress when compared to the nondominant elbow. Therefore, asymmetry of a static valgus stress test alone is typically not sufficient to diagnose an ulnar collateral ligament injury in a throwing athlete.

The milking maneuver has been described as a useful test to assess the functionally more important posterior band of the anterior bundle. This is performed by pulling on the patient's thumb in order to apply valgus stress while the patient's shoulder is forward elevated to 90° and elbow flexed beyond 90°. Pain over the UCL with or without apprehension or instability is considered a positive test and suggestive of UCL injury.

Elbow radiographs should be routinely obtained. In rare cases, an avulsion fracture of the sublime tubercle may be seen in acute-on-chronic cases. Radiographs may show calcification or ossification of the medial ligamentous complex. These findings may be evident in chronic UCL injuries; however, they are rarely seen following an acute injury. Stress radiographs using a standardized elbow valgus stress gadget can be used to assess for possible instability and are considered positive when the medial joint opening is found to be greater than 2.9 mm when compared to the contralateral side. Magnetic resonance (MR) imaging has become the gold standard at confirming a diagnosis of UCL injury. MRA has been found to have a sensitivity of 92 % and a specificity of 100 %. It has also been shown to have the best inter-observer reliability. Recent studies have indicated that MRIs may also be prognostic, as retrospective analysis has shown that a UCL injury with higher T2 signal intensity is less likely to respond to conservative treatment. Recently, ultrasound evaluation has also been reported to have usefulness in the diagnosis of UCL injury. Specifically, the dynamic ultrasound test has been found to be a highly reliable tool in diagnosing laxity of the UCL over time as shown by Nazrian et al. and Ciccotti et al.

TREATMENT

The cornerstone of non-operative treatment for UCL injuries is eliminating the aggravating event (i.e., throwing) for an extended period of time and slowly initiating a course of physical therapy that focuses on maintaining elbow range of motion and strengthening the flexor-pronator musculature. Additionally, strengthening exercises focused on the core and shoulder musculature have been shown to minimize forces across the elbow and optimize neuromuscular control of the extremity. These modalities are often done in concordance with daily icing, anti-inflammatory medication, and bracing. Once the elbow is pain free, a well-supervised, progressive return to throwing may be initiated over a 2–3- month period. When non-operative measures are exhausted and an athlete continues to have significant dysfunction with persistent medial elbow pain that prevents the athlete from returning to a prior activity level, surgical intervention may be indicated.

Surgical reconstruction of the ulnar collateral ligament was first described by Jobe et al. in 1986. This technique involved elevation of the flexor muscles off the medial epicondyle as well as a submuscular transposition of the ulnar nerve. Attachment points of the native UCL were identified and re-approximated with two drill holes in the ulna and three drill holes in the medial epicondyle. Palmaris longus autograft was then passed through the tunnels using a figure-of-eight configuration and sutured back to itself. Since Jobe's initial description, there have been numerous modifications described in the literature. These modifications typically involve differing techniques on dealing with graft fixation, ulnar nerve management, and graft configuration. The most commonly used graft in UCL reconstruction is the palmaris longus autograft; however, other autograft options include gracilis, plantaris, or toe extensor tendon. The senior author's (LSO) preferred surgical management of UCL injuries in the overhead athlete depends on the preoperative evaluation of the behavior of the ulnar nerve. If the athlete does not have a subluxating ulnar nerve, then a muscle splitting surgical approach using a modified docking technique is used. If the athlete has a subluxating ulnar nerve, then the preferred method is to transpose the ulnar nerve and elevate and separate the flexor-pronator muscle group off the UCL without disrupting either structure. In either technique, an ipsilateral palmaris longus tendon is harvested and then used to reconstruct the UCL. Once the appropriate drill holes are placed in the medial epicondyle and proximal ulna, the graft is passed through the ulna and Bdocked^ into the medial epicondyle of the humerus. The drill holes in the ulna are made with a 3.2-mm drill bit for a palmaris longus autograft or a 3.5-mm drill bit for a gracilis autograft. After the graft has been passed through the ulnar bone tunnel, the docking site in the medial epicondyle is made with the aid of a 4.5-mm drill hole and connected by two additional 1.5-mm drill holes (one anteriorly and one posteriorly). One end of the graft is passed through the docking hole, and tension is maintained while the other end of the graft positioned over the medial epicondyle in order to determine the location of suture placement so as not to bottom out on the docking hole. Once a braided nonabsorbable suture has been placed on the appropriate location on the end of the graft, both ends of the graft are docked into the main bone tunnel in the medial epicondyle. Once the elbow is taken through a range of motion and appropriate graft tension is confirmed, the sutures are tied securely over the humeral bone bridge, and the graft is fixed in place while the elbow held in 30° of flexion and the forearm in neutral rotation. Additional sutures may then be used to sew the reconstructed graft back to the native UCL stump, further strengthening the reconstruction.

OUTCOMES

The first successful UCL reconstruction surgery was performed in 1974 by Dr. Frank Jobe, on Los Angeles Dodgers pitcher, Tommy John. Prior to this surgery, a UCL tear was considered to be a career-ending injury. Tommy John's return to baseball in 1976 changed the way this injury was viewed and marked the initiation of an evolution of surgical techniques that would take place over the next 40 years. Dr. Jobe's initial results on baseball pitchers and javelin throwers reported a 63 % success rate, as defined by return to pre-injury or better level of participation in athletic activity. This original surgery, however, was associated with a 32 % complication rate, primarily related to postoperative ulnar neuropathy. The numerous modifications to this procedure that have been described through the years have all focused on minimizing complications and optimizing return to play. A recent systematic review looking at numerous series of UCL reconstruction surgeries with a minimum of 75 % follow-up showed an 83 % success rate. This success rate was defined as a rating of Bexcellent on the Conway-Jobe rating scale. The same review identified several advancements in the original technique that appear to be associated with improved rate of return to prior level of play and decreased complication rate. One of the most significant modifications is the development of the muscle splitting technique as described by Smith et al. The original description of this technique was accompanied by a 0 % ulnar neuropathy rate in their series of 22 patients at 1-year follow-up. With the introduction of the docking technique as described by Rohbrough and Altcheck, Dodson et al. reported a 90 % rate of return to previous level of play for at least 1 year and only a 2 % rate of ulnar neuropathy postoperatively. These results were reconfirmed by Koh et al. who used a modified docking technique and reported a 95 % rate of return to sports at the athlete's previous level of competition for at least 1 year and a 5 % rate of ulnar neuropathy.

Overall, the past 30 years has been marked by an evolution in surgical technique to address UCL injuries. Outcomes have steadily improved and have been estimated to achieve an overall 82 % success rate of excellent results. A more recent study looking specifically atMLB pitchers has shown an 83% return to sport following ulnar collateral ligament reconstruction. Although these results are promising and UCL injury is no longer considered a career-ending injury, highperformance athletes should understand that success rate is not 100 %. Posteromedial impingement Posteromedial impingement was first described in 1983 by Wilson et al. This condition has also become known as valgus extension overload syndrome and is almost exclusively found in overhead-throwing athletes.

An overload of medial tension secondary to extreme repetitive valgus stress may lead to injury and inflammation to the surrounding soft tissue structures of the elbow. Microtrauma to the UCL may occur, leading to subtle valgus instability. This instability will lead to excessive force being transmitted to the lateral and posterior elbow compartments that is most significant in the late cocking and follow-through phases, as the elbow comes into extension. With the continuance of throwing in the setting of subtle instability, shear forces due to a combination of compressive and rotatory forces gradually increase, leading to synovitis and osteophyte formation. Osteophyte formation is hastened as abutment of the olecranon with the olecranon fossa that occurs as the elbow extends. This impingement can lead to worsening pain and posterior synovitis. Increased forces across the articular surface of the elbow then lead to chondromalacia and loose body formation.

Valgus extension overload syndrome

EVALUATION

A thorough history of athletes suffering from valgus extension overload syndrome typically involves a complaint of posterior or posteromedial pain during the follow-through phase of throwing. It is during this final phase of throwing that the elbow extends and the posterior osteophytes impinge. Pain that occurs earlier in the throwing cycle (i.e., late cocking/ early acceleration phase) should raise suspicion for other pathology such as UCL injury. If loose bodies are present, the athlete may also report mechanical symptoms such as locking or catching. Physical examination should focus on the evaluation of range of motion. Posterior osteophytes often lead to loss of terminal extension. In these patients, forced terminal extension may lead to pain. Additionally, Andrews described the Bvalgus extension overload test or the valgus extension snap maneuver. In this test, a moderate valgus stress is applied to the elbow with simultaneous palpation of the posteromedial tip of the olecranon. The elbow is then moved from 30° of flexion to full extension. Pain elicited from this maneuver is considered a positive test. As this condition is caused by repetitive valgus strain, the examiner must also assess for UCL laxity. Imaging of overhead athletes with suspected valgus extension overload syndrome should first include plain radiographs of the elbow. Anteroposterior, lateral, and axial views are typically the views of choice. The axial view has been shown to be helpful in detecting osteophytes on the olecranon or on the borders of the posterior fossa. However, our preference is to obtain a computed tomography (CT) scan. A CT scan may be used to further assess or rule out other bony pathology that could cause similar pain symptoms such as stress fractures or avulsion fractures. Magnetic resonance imaging with or without intra-articular contrast may also be a useful imaging modality in many cases. The sensitivity of the MRI for identifying posterior loose bodies or osteophytes has been found to be 90 %.

TREATMENT

Non-operative treatment of valgus extension overload syndrome consists of an initial period of rest along with a course of ice and anti-inflammatories. Once the initial pain resolves, functional strengthening of the elbow and forearm is initiated with the aid of stretching and isotonic and isometric strengthening. s range of motion and strength improve, strengthening of the flexor-pronator musculature and a supervised throwing program can be progressively initiated. Surgical intervention is indicated if these modalities fail or if the athlete is having significant mechanical symptoms secondary to loose bodies within the elbow joint. The surgical procedure of choice in the overhead athlete that fails conservative treatment of posteromedial impingement is osteophyte excision and exploration for loose bodies. Although this procedure was originally described by Bennet et al. as an open procedure, the current trend is for arthroscopic intervention. Elbow arthroscopy allows visualization of all compartments as well as arthroscopic evaluation of the UCL with an arthroscopic valgus stress test. With arthroscopy, chondromalacia of the ulnohumeral or lateral-sided radiocapitellar joint may be treated with debridement or drilling. Loose body excision and debridement of hypertrophic scar tissue and synovium can also be adequately addressed through the arthroscope. Posterior and posteromedial osteophytes can be easily visualized and debrided to address impingement within the olecranon fossa. Care is taken to debride only enough osteophyte that is needed to allow impingement-free motion. Over-resection has been associated with delayed rupture of the UCL. (Andrews et al.) A crucial portion of the elbow arthroscopy is the intraarticular evaluation of the UCL. An arthroscopic valgus stress test is performed with the elbow in 70° of flexion. If, under direct visualization, medial opening of greater than 1– 2 mm occurs, ulnar collateral ligament insufficiency is suggested. If insufficiency is noted, surgical reconstruction of the UCL must be considered to minimize recurrence and optimize outcome.

OUTCOMES

The results of arthroscopic treatment for symptomatic and recalcitrant valgus extension overload syndrome are variable in the literature. Andrews and Timmerman reported on 56 major league baseball pitchers who underwent arthroscopic posterior olecranon osteophyte excision. There series found a 68 % return to play for at least one season; however, it was associated with a 41 % reoperation rate. They concluded that the incidence of UCL insufficiency in these overhead athletes was likely underestimated and that procedures solely addressing secondary effects of UCL insufficiency (posteromedial osteophytes) without addressing the underlying primary pathology are associated with unsatisfactory results.

More recently, Reddy et al. reviewed 187 elbow arthroscopies. In their series, 51%of patients had posterior olecranon impingement, 31 % were noted to have loose bodies, and 22 % were reported to have findings consistent with degenerative joint disease. Of this cohort, they reported an 85%return to previous level of competition. Their reoperation rate was not reported. It has been hypothesized that these mixed results are likely secondary to an initial void in our understanding of the underlying pathology. Currently, it is unclear whether the removal of posteromedial osteophytes uncovers underlying UCL insufficiency or their excision places the overhead athlete at increased risk of UCL rupture with return to throwing secondary to increased strain on the medial elbow. Long-termfollowup studies that utilize the arthroscopic valgus stress test for intra-articular UCL evaluation will likely be needed to definitively answer this question. Ulnar neuropathy in the overhead athlete Ulnar nerve symptoms are common in the throwing athlete and have been estimated to occur in over 40%of athletes with valgus instability. These symptoms may occur secondary to traction from excessive valgus stress, compression by nearby osteophytes, flexor muscle hypertrophy, or irritation due to subluxation.

Ulnar neuritis

EVALUATION

Throwing athletes with ulnar neuropathy typically complain of paresthesia in the small and ring fingers that occurs during or after throwing. A full motor sensory exam of the upper extremity should be performed with specific attention to hand intrinsic strength and muscle mass. Any weakness or atrophy ompared to the contralateral extremity should be noted and alert the clinician to potential ulnar nerve compression or irritation. Although ulnar nerve compression can typically occur anywhere along the upper extremity, in throwing athletes, it almost exclusively occurs about the elbow. A positive Tinel's sign over the cubital tunnel or just proximal or distal to the tunnel often confirms ulnar neuropathy at the level of the elbow. In these patients, the elbow should be taken through a range of motion and UCL competency should be carefully tested. Palpation of the ulnar nerve during flexion/extension of the elbow should also be performed to rule out ulnar nerve subluxation—a common cause of ulnar neuritis in the overhead athlete.

TREATMENT

Non-operative treatment of ulnar neuritis includes rest, avoidance of inciting activity, and the use of anti-inflammatory medication. Once pain resolves, an interval, supervised, throwing program may be initiated. In patients with ulnar nerve subluxation, the elbow may be splinted for a period of 6 weeks to immobilize the nerve and minimize irritation. When non-operative measures fail to alleviate the symptoms of ulnar neuropathy in the overhead athlete, surgical treatment is indicated. Treatment options typically include in situ ulnar nerve decompression versus ulnar nerve decompression with transposition. The decision to transpose the nerve or perform an in situ decompression should be based on whether or not the ulnar nerve is found to be unstable on preoperative exam or at the time of surgery. Ulnar nerve decompression takes place with a medialbased incision centered over the medial epicondyle. Once the medial antebrachial cutaneous nerve is identified and protected, dissection is taken down to the cubital tunnel and the ulnar nerve is identified. The nerve is then decompressed beginning proximally at the arcade of Struthers and extending distally down to the flexor carpi ulnaris muscle belly origin are is taken to ensure adequate decompression at all the potential sites of compression as described by Amadio et al., including the arcade of Struthers, intermuscular septum, Osborne's fascia, fascia of the flexor carpi ulnaris, and the two heads of the flexor carpi ulnaris as well as the deep aponeurosis of the flexor carpi ulnaris. In athletes who did not demonstrate an unstable ulnar nerve preoperatively, the stability of the ulnar nerve needs to be assessed after the neurolysis to determine its stability. A transposition should be performed if the nerve is felt to be unstable. Subcutaneous transposition is commonly utilized to address the unstable ulnar nerve in the overhead-throwing athlete compared to a submuscular transposition so as not to disrupt the flexor-pronator muscle group that is important for medial elbow stability as a dynamic stabilizer. With submuscular transposition, the flexor origin is elevated off the medial epicondyle and then reattached through drill holes after the nerve is moved anteriorly. In subcutaneous transposition, the nerve is moved anteriorly and rests on top of the flexor origin. It may be held in place by fascial slings that have been created by the flexor fascia distally or the intermuscular septum proximally. Care should be taken that these fascial slings do not create a new area of compression or kinking of the ulnar nerve.

OUTCOMES

Traditionally, authors have advocated for submuscular transposition of the ulnar nerve in the overhead athlete as they believe this better protects the nerve from future direct or indirect trauma. Several of these reports have shown excellent results with high rates of return to play. A potential disadvantage of submuscular transposition is the lengthy rehabilitation period that is required to allow the reattached flexor-pronator origin time to heal. Andrews and Timmerman advocate for anterior subcutaneous ulnar nerve transfer with their report on eight professional baseball players that underwent this procedure. They reported an 88% return to play for at least one season at the professional level. These results were further reinforced by Rettig et al. when they reported a 95 % return to play at an average 12.6 weeks postoperatively in 20 high-level athletes. As previously discussed, ulnar neuritis is often seen in the setting of UCL insufficiency. In this setting, concomitant procedures for UCL reconstruction and ulnar nerve decompression, with or without transposition, are indicated. More recently, Cain et al. looked at 1281 UCL reconstructions. All cases were performed along with an anterior subcutaneous ulnar nerve transposition. In this study, 83 % of athletes returned to the same or higher level of play postoperatively. They reported a 16 % incidence of postoperative ulnar nerve symptoms with anterior subcutaneous transposition. All but one of these cases fully resolved without further intervention by 1 year. Flexor-pronator muscle mass injuries- Much of the dynamic stability about the medial elbow during the throwing cycle is provided by the common flexor-pronator muscle origin. Repetitive valgus stress leads to continued muscle contraction of the common flexor-pronator muscle, which can lead to muscle fatigue and may lead to injury. These injuries typically occur during the acceleration and follow-through phases of the throwing cycle with forceful extension of the elbow and pronation of the forearm. Injuries can range from mild muscular overuse to chronic tendinitis or acute muscle tears.

EVALUATION AND TREATMENT

The overhead athlete with flexor-pronator muscle mass injury typically complains of medial-sided elbow pain during the late cocking or acceleration phase. This is a typical presentation of UCL injury, and so careful examination must be performed in order to differentiate between the two pathologies. Flexor muscle or tendon injury typically demonstrates tenderness just distal to the common tendon origin from the medial epicondyle. UCL injury is noted to have tenderness posterior and distal to the common flexor tendon, along the anterior band of the UCL. The vast majority of flexor-pronator muscle mass injuries respond well to non-operative treatment. This entails rest, anti-inflammatory medication, and physical therapy. Once pain has resolved, a gradual return to throwing may be initiated. For those patients that continue to experience medial pain despite adequate non-operative treatment, the clinician should have suspicion for other, more serious underlying pathology. When imaging and exam confirm an isolated flexor-pronator muscle mass injury, and the patient has exhausted nonoperative easures, surgical side-to-side repair of the tears or re-insertion to the medial epicondyle may be performed as described by Norwood et al.

CONCLUSION

Elbow pain in the overhead-throwing athlete has become more commonplace in recent years. Appropriate diagnosis and management of these patients not only requires a working knowledge of the osseous, ligamentous, nervous, and musculotendinous structures of the medial elbow but also mandates the clinician understand certain biomechanical aspects of the throwing cycle. This will assist a vigilant and thorough clinician with obtaining an accurate diagnosis early on in a patient's symptomatology and potentially improve the chances of successful non-operative treatment. For those athletes who ultimately require surgical intervention, future research aimed at furthering our understanding of the anatomy, biomechanics, and pathophysiology associated with overhead activities will likely lead to continued further improvements in our surgical outcomes.

CHAPTER THREE

OLECRANON BURSITIS

INTRODUCTION

Olecranon bursitis is characterized by an abnormal increase in the volume of fluid within the bursal cavity. The bursal lining is a poorly vascularised synovial membrane that has a low coefficient of friction, thereby allowing the bony olecranon to glide under the skin during flexion and extension of the elbow. This superficial position and limited vascularity makes the olecranon bursa particularly vulnerable to injury and inflammation. It is this limited vascularity that is the proposed reason for infection via a transcutaneous route, rather than via haematogenous spread, even when no obvious wound is present. Staphylococcus aureus predominates as the causative bacteria, with b-haemolytic strep also being common. Of the 150 human bursa, the olecranon is the most commonly affected by an inflammatory process. Despite the frequent presentation of this condition to both primary and secondary care, there is no randomized control data available and, with multiple small number studies often providing conflicting findings, there is currently no consensus on treatment.

Olecranon bursitis, a relatively common condition, is inflammation of the subcutaneous synovial-lined sac of the bursa overlying the olecranon process at the proximal aspect of the ulna. The bursa cushions the olecranon and reduces friction between it and the skin, especially during movement. The superficial location of the bursa, between the ulna and the skin at the posterior tip of the elbow, makes it susceptible to inflammation from acute or repetitive (cumulative) trauma. Less commonly, inflammation results from infection (septic bursitis). Many cases are idiopathic, however.

AETIOLOGY

Initially, it is important to recognize those red flag signs suggesting a neoplastic pathology mimicking a simple olecranon bursitis. Such signs include a rapidly expanding growth, failure of initial treatment, weight loss and prior history of neoplasia. Under these circumstances, appropriate referral, investigation, biopsy and treatment should be undertaken.

The bursa allows the skin to glide freely over the olecranon process, thereby preventing tissue tears. As previously stated, the superficial location of the olecranon bursa makes it susceptible to inflammation from acute or repetitive trauma.

Acute injuries during sports activities can include any action that involves direct or repetitive minor trauma to the posterior elbow (eg, landing on the olecranon process during a fall onto a hard floor or an artificial-turf playing field). Common causes of olecranon bursal inflammation that are unrelated to sports activities include repetitive microtrauma (eg, the elbow constantly rubbing against a table during writing).

Bursal infection, a less common cause of olecranon bursitis, can result from abrasion or laceration at the affected site or from seeding from hematogenous spread via bacteremia. Inflammation can also be cause by a systemic inflammatory process (eg, rheumatoid arthritis) or a crystal-deposition disease (eg, gout, pseudogout). Patients are also at increased risk if they have diabetes mellitus, uremia, a history of intravenous drug abuse, alcohol abuse, or long-term use of steroids.

In patients on long-term hemodialysis treatment, uremia or a mechanical insult (such as resting the posterior elbow during hemodialysis treatment) is thought possibly to cause bursitis. Inflammation of the bursa can also be an adverse effect of the drug sunitinib, which is used to treat patients with renal cell carcinoma.

Larsen et al reported a case of bacillus Calmette-Guérin (BCG) olecranon bursitis developing from disseminated BCG infection, the result of BCG treatment for superficial bladder cancer.

A retrospective study by Schermann et al of olecranon bursitis in the Israel Defense Forces found the condition to be more prevalent in combat units than in noncombat units, with most of the diagnoses being made during those periods of the year, summer and autumn, when training is particularly intensive. The stated that the relatively high number of olecranon bursitis cases diagnosed during those months is probably related to outdoor training that requires crawling and suggested that the use of protective gear could alleviate the problem.

PROGNOSIS

In the absence of infection, most cases of olecranon bursitis respond very well to a series of 1-2 joint aspirations (with or without corticosteroid injection) combined with additional treatment. Some patients may experience recurrence of olecranon bursitis, in which even a relatively minor bump causes a significant effusion to return at this site.

COMPLICATIONS

Complications of olecranon bursitis include progressive or persistent pain with associated difficulty in using the affected upper extremity. Potential complications of aspiration/injection include the following:

- Bleeding
- Bruising
- Allergic reaction (to the corticosteroid)
- Swelling - This may recur, particularly if the patient does not maintain adequate pressure or icing at the site or if an infection was present at the time of the initial aspiration.
- Infection - The clinician should use appropriate techniques, including aseptic techniques, to minimize the chance of iatrogenic infection.
- Persistent drainage through the injection tract.
- Ulnar nerve injury - This theoretically may occur if a medial approach is used for the aspiration/injection.
- Transient elevation of blood glucose levels - This may occur after corticosteroid injection in a diabetic patient.
- Cardiac arrhythmia - This potentially can result from intravascular injection, due to the local anesthetic component.
- Peripheral nerve dysfunction - This is possible if the injection is administered near or within a major nerve.
- Compromised wound healing.
- Gastric, hepatic, and renal adverse effects from NSAIDs and narcotic analgesics.

PATIENT EDUCATION

The patient should be educated regarding olecranon bursitis's diagnosis, causative factors, and treatment plan. The most important aspect of patient education is ensuring that the patient knows to immediately report any signs or symptoms of persistent drainage or infection, particularly if a corticosteroid injection has been given. Diabetic patients should be told that they may experience a transient increase in blood glucose levels. Patients should be informed that a corticosteroid usually does not begin to provide symptomatic improvement until a few days after the injection. Patients should also understand that they may experience a mild, transient increase in symptoms during the window of time when the local anesthetic has worn off but the steroids have not begun to have a therapeutic effect.

PRESENTATION

History

Patient history may include the following findings:

Focal swelling at the posterior elbow is usually noticed by the patient

The patient may report pain at the affected site, although sometimes the swelling is painless, especially in noninflammatory, aseptic bursitis. Pain often is exacerbated by pressure, such as when the patient leans on the elbow or when the patient rubs the elbow against a table while writing with the ipsilateral hand or with associated prolonged elbow flexion over 90°. Chronic, recurrent swelling usually is not tender; swelling may have gradual (mostly due to a chronic cause) or acute/sudden (due to trauma or infection/inflammation) onset. Frequent bumping of the swollen elbow may occur because the elbow protrudes further than normal.

The patient may report a history of isolated trauma (eg, contusion) or repetitive microtrauma (such as constant rubbing of the elbow against a table while writing). The onset may be sudden if the condition is secondary to infection or acute trauma. The onset may be gradual if olecranon bursitis is secondary to chronic irritation

PHYSICAL EXAMINATION

The most classic finding in olecranon bursitis is posterior elbow swelling that is often fluctuant and that is very clearly demarcated, appearing as a goose egg over the olecranon process. Other findings in olecranon bursitis include the following:

- The affected site may be tender to palpation; pain is variable; severe pain is often due to a traumatic or infectious cause; pain with pressure on the tip of the elbow may interfere with sleep.
- The area may be warm and red, particularly with infection
- Skin inspection may reveal abrasion or contusion if trauma recently occurred
- Vital signs may reveal fever, but generally only with advanced infection.
- Elbow range of motion (ROM) usually is normal, but occasionally the end range of elbow flexion is slightly limited because of pain or, in

chronic cases, due to bursal thickening; this decreased ROM may interfere with performance of basic activities of daily living, such as dressing, bathing, and grooming.
- Patients with systemic inflammatory processes (eg, rheumatoid arthritis) or a crystal deposition disease (eg, gout, pseudogout) may reveal evidence of focal inflammation at other sites or extending distally in the forearm if there is an associated cellulitis. Upon inspection of the elbow, rheumatoid nodules may be found in patients with rheumatoid arthritis; firm "bumps" or "lumps", due to residual scar tissue, may be felt as swelling recedes, especially when the elbow is bumped. Sensation should not be impaired, distal pulses should be intact, and other joints should not be affected.

DIAGNOSTIC CONSIDERATIONS

If there is a history of trauma, elbow pain during active or passive ROM may increase the clinician's suspicion of fracture of the olecranon process. Other conditions to consider in the differential diagnosis of olecranon bursitis include the following:

- Crystalline inflammatory arthropathy (eg, gout, pseudogout)
- Fracture of the olecranon process of the ulna
- Synovial cyst of the elbow joint
- Olecranon traction osteophyte (with or without avulsion)
- Olecranon spur (usually without joint effusion)
- Presence of infection (the most important consideration)
- Triceps tendinitis/tear
- Lipoma
- Elbow and Forearm Overuse Injuries
- Gout and Pseudogout
- Olecranon Fractures
- Rheumatoid Arthritis
- Triceps Tendon Avulsion

WORKUP

Approach Considerations

Usually, laboratory studies are necessary only if the clinician suspects that an underlying condition is present. It is necessary to check for infection (complete blood count [CBC], including a differential count of the white blood cells [WBCs]). Tests should also be run for rheumatoid factor, the erythrocyte sedimentation rate, and the C-reactive protein level, in order to assess for rheumatoid arthritis. The uric acid level should be checked in order to assess for gout.

Gram Stain

If infection is suspected (due to the presence of fever, redness, previous puncture wounds, or cellulitis), the olecranon bursa should be aspirated and the fluid sent for culture, for a cell count (WBCs, red blood cells [RBCs]), and for immediate Gram staining for bacteria. If the Gram stain is positive for bacteria, antibiotics should be started immediately and no corticosteroids should be injected into the bursa.

However, even if the Gram stain is negative or initially unavailable, withholding corticosteroid injection and starting antibiotics may seem indicated based on the mechanism of injury (eg, abrasion or puncture), physical examination findings suggestive of infection (eg, fever, significant local redness and warmth), or the gross appearance of the aspirate (eg, turbid, purulent).

WBC Count and Bacterial Culture

WBC count

The leukocyte count can help to determine whether the fluid is infectious or merely inflammatory. Within synovial aspirates, WBC counts are assessed as follows:

- Normal - Less than 200/μL
- Non-inflammatory - 200-2000/μL
- Indication of inflammation - Count in the range of 2000-100,000/μL
- Indication of a septic condition - Count greater than 100,000/μL

Bacterial culture

Bacterial culture and sensitivity testing of the aspirate can be performed to ensure the relevant bacteria are sensitive to the chosen antibiotic. These results can guide the modification of antibiotics in cases of bacterial infection.

OTHER FINDINGS

After an acute injury, blood may be found within the aspirate, indicating a hemorrhagic bursitis.

Ultrasonography

The use of ultrasonography has been shown to be extremely effective in the diagnosis of olecranon bursitis and other soft-tissue lesions in the olecranon area by rapidly demonstrating the presence of effusions, synovial proliferation, loose bodies, increased blood flow consistent with inflammation, tendonitis with calcifications, and other indications of bursitis.

Magnetic resonance imaging

In atypical cases, a magnetic resonance imaging (MRI) study may be indicated to help exclude concomitant pathology, such as a stress fracture, triceps tendinopathy or tear, or the rare case of osteomyelitis/abscess or tumor, especially if there is a long history of septic bursitis or to evaluate an unusual mass seen on plain radiographs.

Bursal Aspiration

The olecranon bursa can be aspirated using a long 18-gauge needle that is inserted after sterile skin preparation, using a circular motion with an antibacterial solution (after determining no applicable allergies exist) and appropriate local infiltration with a suitable agent, such as 1% lidocaine, using sterile technique to avoid secondary infection and a 27- to 30-gauge needle to make a skin wheal over the lateral bursa. The 18-gauge needle is attached to a 10-mL syringe and inserted into the dependent area of the bursa through a posterolateral approach, via an oblique needle angle or zigzag approach.

As opposed to a direct, perpendicular approach that is used for most joint aspirations, this technique creates a longer needle tract through the skin and subcutaneous layers, thus minimizing the risk of fistula formation. The medial approach to the olecranon bursa should be avoided, since a misdirected needle could damage the ulnar nerve. Aspiration of bursal contents is continued until the bursal site is flat. The needle is then withdrawn and the wound dressed with adhesive sterile bandage and the elbow wrapped with a compressive dressing. Active elbow range of motion should be restricted for about 2 days post injection.

If any cloudy fluid is aspirated, it should be sent for immediate Gram stain, leukocyte count, culture, and antibiotic sensitivity testing. No corticosteroids should be given until these tests prove negative. Aspiration can also be therapeutic, because it relieves the swelling. If cultures of aspirated fluid are negative and fluid recurs, the bursal aspiration can be repeated and, if sterile on culture, corticosteroids can be considered for joint injection.

If the clinician is confident that no infection is present, corticosteroid injection can be considered (for instance, immediately after aspiration of the fluid). In the absence of a traumatic etiology, consideration should be given to analyzing the aspirated fluid for infection and crystals. When aspiration/injection is performed, aseptic techniques should be used to minimize the chance of causing iatrogenic infection. Septic olecranon bursitis due to Mycobacterium smegmatis has been reported after intrabursal steroid injection.

Trauma

Most commonly, olecranon bursitis is a non-infective, post-traumatic, inflammatory response to repetitive, minor trauma. Historically, this has prompted the introduction of a variety of pseudonyms, including 'students elbow' and 'plumbers elbow'. An isolated traumatic event can also initiate the inflammatory cascade but, under these circumstances, an underlying fracture must be excluded. In the absence of blunt trauma, a penetrating foreign body must also be considered as a potential cause of a traumatic bursitis.

Medical conditions

Olecranon bursitis is known to be associated with common medical conditions, either directly or as a consequence of immunosuppression secondary to therapeutic intervention. Relatively common conditions with a direct association include diabetes mellitus, gout, rheumatoid arthritis, alcoholism and HIV. Some conditions, which include inflammatory bowel disease, respiratory disease and polymyalgia rheumatica/giant cell arteritis, are often treated with immunosuppressant therapy, and this will increase the risk of developing infective bursitis.

Diagnostics

The list of known causes and associated risk factors summarized above is neither summative, nor exhaustive, although early discrimination of septic from aseptic bursitis has been demonstrated to impact upon the duration of treatment required. Unfortunately, there is accepted difficulty in confirming an infective cause on history and examination alone. Confirmation with aspiration and urgent gram stain and culture can be considered as the gold standard because false positive rates are low provided a suitable aseptic technique is followed.

Other proposed observations and tests have provided a wealth of conflicting evidence, mirroring the frequent overlap between septic and aseptic causes. Swelling, erythema and tenderness, with preserved elbow movement, are universal common features. Fever is present in up to 77% of septic cases and erythema present in 63–100%; therefore, both are only moderately sensitive for infection. Analysis of bursal aspirate is suggested by many and common tests include differential white cell count, comparative glucose concentration and protein levels. When serum glucose is compared with aspirate glucose concentration, a >50% disparity is diagnostic for infection. This test in isolation, however, has been partially discredited, with a false negative rate of 9% being reported. Protein and complement levels showed no statistically significant difference and have low predictive value. Leukocytosis greater than 10,000mm3 is likely diagnostic for sepsis, however, septic aspirate cell counts have been reported from 690 cells/mm3 to 79,400 cells/mm3[1] and non-infective cases were found to range from 50 cells/mm3 to 3450 cells/mm3. This has resulted in false negative reports in up to 12.5% of cases in one study[1] and 31% in another.

A predominance of polymorphs within the aspirate of greater than 50% has been shown as a reliable feature in identifying infection. Monocytes predominate in non-infective samples, comprising >50% of the cell count.

It is worth noting the findings of Hassell et al. who reported a case of seven patients with rheumatoid associated olecranon bursitis. They found aspirate cell concentrations in keeping with septic bursitis; however, all were culture and Gram-stain negative in the absence of antibiotics. Promising results were demonsrated with the sclerosing action of intrabursal tetracycline for rheumatoid bursitis, without the skin atrophy, secondary infections and sinus formation that have been reported as a result of steroid injection. Given the lack of a single highly sensitive and specific test, a detailed history to identify general and specific risk factors focuses on the patient's occupation, hobbies, medical history, medication, family history and recent trauma. Recurrent or nonresolving olecranon bursitis is of particular importance, raising suspicion of retained foreign body, antimicrobial resistance or incorrect diagnosis. Systemic symptoms should be explored, including fevers, anorexia, lethargy, weight loss and night-sweats, which are more suggestive of an infective (or rarely malignant) origin. A thorough general examination of the patient should be followed by specific examination of the affected area and contralateral elbow. Quayle and Robinson reported a case series of olecranon process excisions for non-infective bursitis, where the patients had either an olecranon spur or abnormally prominent olecranon. A 100% cure rate was achieved. The examiner focuses on the size of the swelling, its consistency (soft, firm, hard), fluctuancy, associated erythema, skin temperature, any lymphadenopathy and the characteristics of movement in the elbow joint: specifically range and pain. It is worth noting that our experience mirrors the documented consensus that elbow movement is preserved in bursitis, as opposed to the restriction associated with septic arthritis.

Investigations are preferably performed prior to antibiotic therapy and should include baseline observations, plain film radiographs of the elbow and basic

blood tests, including full blood count; urea and electrolytes; calcium, uric acid, glucose levels; and inflammatory markers such as C-reactive protein and erythrocyte sedimentation rate. The value of blood cultures has been debated, with culture positive rates of 4%, 19% and 30%. Clearly, it would be sensible to reason that, in the presence of systemic features of infection, a bacteraemia is more likely to be diagnosed from blood culture.

Wherever practicable, prior to the administration of antibiotics, needle aspiration of the bursa should be performed cautiously. An aseptic technique will provide a sample for urgent microscopy, culture and sensitivity, at the same time as providing pain relief by reducing the bursal pressure. Violation of the elbow joint by the needle should be avoided to prevent secondary iatrogenic septic arthritis. Ultrasound guidance may be used to assist accuracy. A differential white cell count and determination of glucose levels is also advocated because these are helpful predictors of infection in the absence of a positive Gram stain or culture, as described above. Further imaging with magnetic resonance has been described previously as a sensitive negative predictor of infective bursitis. The absence of bursal and soft tissue enhancement is reported as a reliable indicator of non-infective bursitis, whereas its presence is nonspecific and can be present in up to 76% of cases of any cause.

WORKUP

Usually, laboratory studies are necessary only if the clinician suspects that an underlying condition is present. If infection is suspected (due to the presence of fever, redness, previous puncture wounds, or cellulitis), the olecranon bursa should be aspirated and the fluid sent for culture, for a cell count (white blood cells [WBCs], red blood cells [RBCs]), and for immediate Gram staining for bacteria.

Tests should also be run for rheumatoid factor, the erythrocyte sedimentation rate, and the C-reactive protein level, in order to assess for rheumatoid arthritis. The uric acid level should be checked in order to assess for gout.

Plain radiographs of the elbow should be performed to assess for a possible olecranon fracture if significant trauma occurred or if an avulsed osteophyte is present at the triceps insertion into the olecranon, which is fairly common.

The use of ultrasonography has been shown to be extremely effective in the diagnosis of olecranon bursitis and other soft-tissue lesions in the olecranon area by rapidly demonstrating the presence of effusions, synovial proliferation, loose bodies, increased blood flow consistent with inflammation, tendonitis with calcifications, and other indications of bursitis.

In atypical cases, a magnetic resonance imaging (MRI) study may be indicated to help exclude concomitant pathology, such as a stress fracture, triceps tendinopathy or tear, or the rare case of osteomyelitis/abscess or tumor.

MANAGEMENT

In general, physical and occupational therapy are not needed for the treatment of olecranon bursitis. In some cases of nonseptic bursitis, however, the physician may recommend a course of physical or occupational therapy to speed recovery time. In the absence of infection, most cases of olecranon bursitis respond very well to a series of 1-2 joint aspirations (with or without corticosteroid injection) combined with additional treatment.

Oral nonsteroidal anti-inflammatory drugs (NSAIDs) can help to reduce the pain and inflammation of olecranon bursitis, but these products probably should be avoided if joint aspiration reveals a hemorrhagic bursitis. Injectable corticosteroid can be beneficial in cases in which the history, physical examination, and joint aspiration do not raise a significant suspicion of infection.

Usually, no surgical intervention is required in cases of olecranon bursitis. If the patient's condition becomes severe and does not respond to conservative treatment, however, bursectomy may be indicated. If surgical intervention is required, endoscopic olecranon bursal excision is an effective alternative to open incision in either aseptic or septic cases. Endoscopic outcomes are excellent and can minimize wound-healing problems.

TREATMENT OPTIONS AND COMPLICATIONS

Non-infective

Most commonly, the bursitis will be inflammatory and non-infective. Under these circumstances, symptomatic treatment with elevation, splintage, ice and anti-inflammatories is regarded as the option of choice, although we acknowledge that most do not require elevation in a sling. Routine aspiration and injection of non-infective bursitis with steroid and local anaesthetic has been advocated1 as an appropriate treatment to shorten the natural history; however, Smith et al. oppose this view based on work by Sö derquist and Hedströ m who reported a 10% risk of infection by contamination.

Given the controversy, we have reviewed the two studies that have reported results obtained after steroid injection. Weinstein et al. reported a group of 47 confirmed cases of non-infected olecranon bursitis where all were aspirated but only 25 were infiltrated with corticosteroid. This infiltration was performed 7 days post initial aspiration after sample sterility had been confirmed. A reduction in symptom duration was statistically significant for the steroid group compared to the control group. There were, however, complications associated with the steroid group, with two re-presenting with septic bursitis and five suffering from overlying skin atrophy. Smith et al. subsequently reported a controlled and blinded, prospective trial where the outcomes of 42 aseptic olecranon bursae were divided between four treatment groups. Group 1 received infiltrated steroid with oral nonsteroidal anti-inflammatory drugs (NSAID). Group 2 received infiltrated steroid but with a placebo oral agent. Group 3 received only NSAID and group 4 received only an oral placebo agent. The study failed to demonstrate a statistically significant reduction in symptom duration when adding NSAIDs to the treatment regimen. Infiltrated corticosteroid did, however, show a statistically significant reduction in symptom duration. Furthermore, there were no cases of secondary septic bursitis or skin atrophy reported. Given this evidence, it would appear that NSAIDs may only be helpful for symptomatic relief, whereas corticosteroids, although effective, present a risk of secondary infection and should therefore be used with caution. Where a large and painful bursitis is clinically diagnosed as inflammatory, we will often aspirate in anticipation of beneficial pressure relief. A sample is sent for culture but it is not our practice to inject steroid. When the aetiology is secondary to a known medical pathology and treatment for both the known pathology and bursitis is combined, there is no published evidence to confirm a reduction in the duration of the associated bursitis. It would appear logical, however, and there might be ethical difficulties related to withholding treatment as part of a controlled study. Where there is non-infective bursitis in the presence of an olecranon spur, it is popular opinion that operative excision of the spur can significantly reduce the risk of recurrence, with two small studies reporting success.

Infective

For those less common episodes of infective olecranon bursitis, many treatment options have been proposed. Ho and Su have provided a classification system where clinical signs denote whether a bursitis is mild, moderate or severe.

Mild disease: local inflammation with no systemic signs.

Moderate: significant local inflammation with mild systemic signs.

Severe: intense peri-bursal cellulitis with infected wound with systemic signs, including pyrexia or rigors, or a serum leukocytosis >10,000/mm3.

Importantly, this classification system was devised for observing the duration of antibiotics required to achieve sterility of infected bursal aspirates. The study by Ho et al. specifically excluded patients with 'underlying host defects, such as diabetes mellitus, renal or hepatic disease, underlying malignant disease or rheumatic disease because they are 'more prone to infection and may not respond in the same manner'. This is supported by Garcia-Porrua et al. who demonstrated a longer antibiotic duration was necessary for immunocompromised patients. Given the common association between infected bursitis and co-existing medical conditions, a modification to the Ho–Su classification is proposed, where the presence of co-morbidity likely to affect healing or immune response, increases the severity by one level within the Ho–Su classification. Proposed treatment options are sub-classified as to whether they are performed acutely, or as a delayed procedure following antibiotic therapy. Significant swelling with pointing is considered an indication for incision and drainage, only once attempted aspiration has failed because of loculation. A large retrospective series reviewing the recurrence rates in 237 episodes of infected olecranon bursitis was performed by Perez et al. They found single stage acute bursectomy to be associated with increased recurrence rates compared to multistage open procedures with delayed primary closure. Their study included a 91% acute bursectomy rate (olecranon and prepatella), 41% of which were single stage; however, no information was provided on wound healing duration or complications.

Unfortunately, there are no randomized comparative studies comparing outcomes after acute multistage bursectomy with delayed single stage procedures.

Degree et al. reported a retrospective review of 37 cases of open bursectomy for chronic bursitis. Patients with a gouty or rheumatoid cause were excluded from the study. Some 43% healed without complication, 27% had delayed healing with excessive exudate and 22% suffered recurrence, 50% of whom required further intervention.

Antibiotic duration and administration sparks controversy. Some have advocated outpatient treatment with prolonged oral antibiotics, with or without

percutaneous needle aspiration, whereas others have described immobilization and antibiotics, or hospitalization with surgical drainage or suction irrigation. Furthermore, there is considerable variation between suggested antibiotic protocols, with some advocating up to 4 weeks of intravenous antibiotics in non-operative management. Where operative intervention is employed, adjuvant therapy regimens describe short intravenous courses, followed by oral treatment for up to 2 weeks. In mild cases of infective bursitis, several studies advocate needle aspiration before commencing antibiotics as an outpatient; however, differentiating between mild and more severe cases is open to error, despite no cases of inter-observer error in the original study. Treatment failure rates of between 9% and 32% for mild bursitis, and 48% to 51% for severe bursitis, are reported. It has been suggested that failure to intervene surgically is the most potent independent risk factor for recurrence (14.6% versus 80%), although, without the evidence provided by a large number randomized control trial, it is inappropriate to advocate surgery for all. This suggestion was proposed with adjuvant treatment with either a short or long course of antibiotics. Following a retrospective analysis of 343 episodes of severe infective bursitis requiring hospitalization (237 olecranon, 106 patellae), the following conclusions were drawn;

One-stage bursectomy and closure reduced in-hospital stay by 4 days. Intravenous antibiotics were not required in patients with normal gut function because there was no significant reduction in infection duration with intravenous adjuvant antibiotics. Recurrence rates were not improved with a more than 7-day antibiotic course. Bacteraemia was identified in only 4% of patients. The only independent risk factor for recurrence in postoperative patients was immunosuppression. Recurrence rates secondary to immunosuppression were unaffected by treatment modification. Within the umbrella of 'surgical excision', we include the techniques of arthroscopic versus traditional open procedures, with arthroscopy gaining merit based on reduced theoretical risk of wound complications. We acknowledge that the arthroscopic approach is quite uncommon and, once again, there is no controlledtrial data to support this, although multiple, small number case series report few complications for bursectomy at the olecranon and patella. The feared complications in open excision are wound dehiscence, chronic sinus and skin necrosis as a result of the watershed midline blood supply. Arthroscopic techniques aim to avoid this with port sites located distant from the midline.

Open drainage is generally undertaken for those cases that (i) have an obvious, fluctuant collection, which is either felt unlikely to or has failed to respond to antibiotics, and (ii) where the patient is clearly systemically unwell secondary to the infective process.

Once the infection has settled, and particularly when a history of recurrent bursitis is present, an interval bursectomy is undertaken. Occasionally, under these circumstances, the bursa is no longer obvious and, to delineate its boundaries, our practice is to inflate with saline at the start of the procedure, usually 5mL. If the skin is of good quality, then a midline incision can be made, although often it is densely scarred to the bursal surface. In attempting to dissect between the layers, the tissue is often compromised, resulting in wound dehiscence, which may require further surgery or prolonged outpatient dressing therapy. In an effort to avoid this and because of the surplus tissue often present, an ellipse of skin can be taken, thereby allowing dissection through higher quality tissue. The wound is then far less likely to fail. Where a bony spur is present, this is usually excised simultaneously. At closure, the elliptical incision comes together to provide a well vascularized midline scar.

Approach Considerations

The patient's physical condition and history should be taken into account when administering treatment for olecranon bursitis, as in the following cases:

- Pregnant patient - Aspiration of the bursa and corticosteroid injection can be performed during pregnancy; oral nonsteroidal anti-inflammatory drugs (NSAIDs) should be avoided.

- Elderly patient with history of side effects from NSAIDs - It is necessary to be cautious when using NSAIDs in elderly patients; cyclo-oxygenase-2 (COX-2) inhibitors may be indicated.
- Patient with diabetes - Some patients with diabetes may experience a transient elevation in blood glucose levels after corticosteroid injection.

In general, physical and occupational therapy are not needed for the treatment of olecranon bursitis. In some cases of nonseptic bursitis, however, the physician may recommend a course of physical or occupational therapy to speed recovery time. Usually, no surgical intervention is required in cases of olecranon bursitis. If the patient's condition becomes severe and does not respond to conservative treatment, however, bursectomy may be indicated. Based on a literature review, Baumbach et al suggested that even in cases of septic olecranon bursitis, the evidence supports the initial use of conservative treatment rather than immediate bursectomy. They state that only patients with severe, refractory, chronic/recurrent olecranon bursitis should be treated via incision, drainage, or bursectomy. (They came to the same conclusions for prepatellar bursitis as well.)

If surgical intervention is required in olecranon bursitis, endoscopic olecranon bursal excision is an effective alternative to open incision in either aseptic or septic cases. Endoscopic outcomes are excellent and can minimize wound-healing problems.

A study by Ogilvie-Harris and Gilbart demonstrated that endoscopic bursal resection relieves pain symptoms and typically gives satisfactory results in patients with chronic olecranon bursitis.

A study by Meric et al also reported good results from endoscopic bursectomy, for either prepatellar or olecranon bursitis. The 49 patients in the study, including 30 with olecranon bursitis and 19 with prepatellar bursitis, were treated endoscopically (25 patients) or with open bursectomy (24 patients). At followup, the endoscopic group scored 8.5 on a patient satisfaction questionnaire, compared with 5.3 by the open surgery group.

A study by Uçkay et al suggested that for adult patients with moderate to severe septic olecranon bursitis, the rate of wound dehiscence is lower with onestage bursectomy than with a two-stage approach to the procedure. The investigators found that 1 out of 66 patients in the one-stage group experienced wound dehiscence, compared with 9 out of 64 in the two-stage group.

PREVENTION

- A compressive elbow sleeve (eg, a neoprene or elastic sleeve) may help to prevent the bursal fluid from reaccumulating after aspiration, but the application of excessive pressure over the elbow should be avoided.
- Avoiding further trauma to the olecranon bursa is the key to recovery and prevention of recurrence.
- Consider use of elbow pads to cushion the elbow.
- For cases of olecranon bursitis in which there is repeated recurrence, consider use of a posterior plaster splint to limit elbow motion for 1-2 weeks following aspiration.
- For severely recalcitrant cases, consider referral to an orthopedic surgeon for possible bursal excision.

Monitoring
The patient should return for reevaluation within approximately 2 weeks after treatment. At that time, assessment should be made regarding reaccumulation of fluid, persistent drainage, and signs of infection.

Activity
The athlete with olecranon bursitis may be expected to return to play without restrictions after he/she has demonstrated resolution of symptoms and of any positive physical examination findings (eg, swelling, tenderness to palpation) and has shown adequate performance in sports-specific practice drills without recurrence of symptoms or physical examination findings.

Aspiration
As previously mentioned, in the absence of infection most cases of olecranon bursitis respond very well to a series of 1-2 joint aspirations (with or without corticosteroid injection) combined with additional treatment.

A retrospective study by Weinstein and colleagues showed that in 47 patients with traumatic olecranon bursitis, almost all cases resolved via aspiration, with or without intrabursal glucocorticoid injection. In the 25 patients who did receive glucocorticoid injection (20 mg of triamcinolone) in addition to bursal aspiration, the bursitis resolved much more rapidly than it did in the other patients, usually within 1 week. However, there seemed to be an association between the glucocorticoid injections and the development of complications, such as infection and skin atrophy.

A study by Kim et al reported that in the treatment of nonseptic olecranon bursitis, no difference in efficacy was found between the uses of aspiration, the use of aspiration combined with steroid injections, and the use of compression bandaging combined with nonsteroidal anti-inflammatory drugs (NSAIDs), at 4- week follow-up. The investigators cautioned, however, that the study, which involved 83 patients, was powered to identify no less than a 30% difference between the three treatments, which means that if a smaller difference in efficacy existed, it may not have been detected.

Pharmacologic Therapy

Oral NSAIDs can help to reduce the pain and inflammation of olecranon bursitis, but these products probably should be avoided if joint aspiration reveals a hemorrhagic bursitis. Injectable corticosteroid can be beneficial in cases in which the history, physical examination, and joint aspiration do not raise a significant suspicion of infection.

Focal corticosteroid injection may be an option, but only if the clinician is confident that no local infection is present. The decision as to whether the patient should be treated with empiric antibiotics depends on the perceived likelihood of infection, as indicated by patient history, physical examination, and analysis of the bursal aspirate.

In a study of 343 episodes of infectious bursitis, including 237 episodes of olecranon bursitis and 106 of patellar bursitis, Perez et al found that 7 days or less of antibiotic treatment was as effective as antibiotic therapy lasting from 8 days to more than 2 weeks. The investigators also found that short-course antibiotic therapy was not associated with a recurrence of bursitis.

Injection technique

The injection should be on the lateral side of the elbow, so as to avoid the ulnar nerve. The target injection site is the soft-tissue center of the triangle formed by the lateral olecranon, the head of the radius, and the lateral epicondyle. As with most injections, the physician should first aspirate to ensure that the needle is not in a blood vessel and then inject using a slow, but consistent, pressure. Corticosteroids should never be injected into a site that appears to be infected or through skin that appears to be infected.

Physical Therapy

As previously mentioned, although physical and occupational therapy are generally not needed for olecranon bursitis, in some nonseptic cases the physician may recommend a course of physical or occupational therapy to speed recovery time. Individuals who exhibit olecranon bursitis often are advised to apply the RICE (rest, ice, compression, elevation) method of treatment. Icing of the posterior elbow for 15-20 minutes at a time, several times daily, is recommended during the acute period (2-5 days).

Physical therapy modalities (eg, phonophoresis, electrical stimulation) also may be helpful in further reducing pain and inflammation, although these modalities are not necessary for most patients.

The therapist can also complete patient education and present compensatory strategies for resting the involved upper extremity while healing takes place. For the patient who undergoes bursal excision (bursectomy), physical therapy may be recommended postoperatively for regaining or maintaining the elbow's ROM and strength.

Consultations

- Consultation with a physiatrist (physical medicine and rehabilitation physician) or with another qualified musculoskeletal specialist may be considered by physicians without the training, comfort, or procedural office supplies necessary for joint aspiration.
- Consultation with a rheumatologist may be helpful if the clinical findings are consistent with inflammatory arthropathy.
- Consultation with an orthopedic surgeon is required if a fracture is present, if the patient has a very severe case of recalcitrant bursitis that requires excision (bursectomy), or if incision and drainage are required for septic bursitis.

MEDICATION
Medication Summary

Medications are used in cases of olecranon bursitis primarily to decrease pain and inflammation. Thus, the most commonly used medications are oral NSAIDs and focal corticosteroid injection, in conjunction with the rest of the rehabilitation plan.

As previously stated, however, oral NSAIDs probably should be avoided if joint aspiration reveals a hemorrhagic bursitis. Injectable corticosteroid can be beneficial in cases in which the history, physical examination, and joint aspiration do not raise a significant suspicion for infection.

Empiric antibiotic selection is based on the suspected source of the microorganisms (local invasion by skin flora via puncture or abrasion, or hematogenous spread from a primary infection at another body site). Initial antibiotic selection is also directed by the results of the Gram stain of the aspirate.

Antibiotic treatment may start with a broad-spectrum antibiotic; then, when the culture and sensitivity test results are available, the antibiotic regimen may be modified as appropriate.

Nonsteroidal Anti-Inflammatory Drugs (NSAIDs)

NSAIDs can help to decrease pain and inflammation. Various oral NSAIDs can be used. The choice of an agent is largely based on its adverse-effect profile, as well as on convenience (how frequently doses must be taken to achieve adequate analgesic and anti-inflammatory effects), patient preferences, and cost.

Although increased treatment cost can be a negative factor, the incidence of costly and potentially fatal gastrointestinal (GI) bleeds is clearly less with cyclooxygenase- 2 (COX-2) inhibitors than with traditional NSAIDs. Ongoing analysis of cost avoidance in cases of GI bleeds will further define the populations that will find COX-2 inhibitors to be the most beneficial.

Ibuprofen (Motrin, Advil, Addaprin, Caldolor)

Ibuprofen is the drug of choice for mild to moderate pain. It inhibits inflammatory reactions and pain by decreasing prostaglandin synthesis. Many doses are available, either with or without a prescription.

Celecoxib (Celebrex)

Celecoxib inhibits primarily COX-2. COX-2 is considered an inducible isoenzyme, induced during pain and inflammatory stimuli. Inhibition of COX-1 may contribute to NSAID GI toxicity. At therapeutic concentrations, the COX-1 isoenzyme is not inhibited; thus, GI toxicity may be decreased. Seek the lowest dose of celecoxib for each patient.

Naproxen (Anaprox, Naprelan, Naprosyn)

Naproxen is used for the relief of mild to moderate pain. It inhibits inflammatory reactions and pain by decreasing the activity of cyclo-oxygenase (COX), which is responsible for prostaglandin synthesis.

Ketoprofen

Ketoprofen is used for the relief of mild to moderate pain and inflammation. Small doses are indicated initially in patients with small body size, elderly patients, and persons with renal or liver disease. Doses of over 75 mg do not increase therapeutic effects. Administer high doses with caution, and closely observe the patient for response.

Corticosteroids

In contrast to the widespread, systemic distribution of an oral anti-inflammatory drug, a local corticosteroid injection can achieve focal placement of a potent anti-inflammatory agent at the site of maximal tenderness or inflammation. A variety of corticosteroid preparations are available for injection. Commonly, the corticosteroid is mixed with a local anesthetic agent prior to injection. Various local anesthetic agents also are available.

Methylprednisolone (Depo-Medrol, Solu-Medrol, Medrol, A-Methapred)

Corticosteroids, such as methylprednisolone, are commonly used for local injections of bursae or joints to provide a local anti-inflammatory effect while minimizing some of the GI and other risks of systemic medications. Methylprednisolone decreases inflammation by suppressing the migration of polymorphonuclear leukocytes and reversing increased capillary permeability.

Dexamethasone (Baycadron)

Dexamethasone may reduce steroid hormone production. It decreases immune reactions. Dexamethasone provides a local anti-inflammatory effect while

minimizing some of the gastrointestinal and other risks associated with systemic medications.

CHAPTER FOUR

ROTATOR-CUFF INJURY

INTRODUCTION
Shoulder pain results in over three million visits to physicians each year. Of these visits, rotator cuff disease is the most common cause. Yamamoto et al. showed 20.7% of 1366 shoulders had full-thickness rotator cuff tears in the general population with the biggest risk factors being age, dominant arm, and history of trauma. Even with advances in surgical management of rotator cuff injuries, recurrent tears of large or massive repairs remain a problem, in some cases ranging from 13 to 94%. It is imperative that patients not only have extremely skilled surgical care but a knowledgeable and experienced physical therapist to help guide their post-operative progression. Successful treatment of rotator cuff repair relies on constant communication between the surgical and rehabilitation staff. The ultimate goal of post-operative rehabilitation after rotator cuff repair is to relieve pain and restore range of motion as well as prior levels of function. In order to properly treat this group of patients, a sound understanding of anatomy, biomechanics, and evidence-based exercise progression are essential.

ANATOMY
The rotator cuff is composed of a group of four muscles and tendons that surround the shoulder. These include the supraspinatus, infraspinatus, subscapularis, and teres minor which function to assist in glenohumeral (GH) elevation and rotation. When working together, this group of muscles creates force vectors which provide dynamic stability to the GH joint by maintaining centralization of the humeral head within the glenoid fossa. The supraspinatus plays an important role in GH joint stability and is responsible for initiating abduction and rotation of the joint as well as compression at lower elevation angles. The infraspinatus and teres minor make up the posterior rotator cuff and are largely responsible for external rotation of the shoulder as well as providing an inferior compression force

of the humeral head in the glenoid, which helps minimize subacromial impingement. The subscapularis works to internally rotate the shoulder and provide compression as well as anterior stability. When functioning properly, the rotator cuff complex allows for GH movement with stability; however, if the rotator cuff becomes damaged or torn through injury or disease, dysfunction may occur.

COMPLICATIONS

Although surgical techniques have improved and postoperative rehab techniques have advanced, complication management should be addressed. In a recent systematic review, the most frequently encountered complication was re-rupture or re-tear of the repair, ranging from 11 and 95%, followed by stiffness and hardware-related complications which ranged from 1.5 to 11.1%. Numerous authors reported stiffness as the most common complication ranging from 2.7 to 15%. Other reported complications include nerve injury, reflex sympathetic dystrophy, infection, hardware failure, deep venous thrombosis, and complications related to anesthesia. Although these other complications have been reported, postoperative shoulder stiffness remains one of the most common issues and one that clinicians should be cautious of during treatment.

REHABILITATION GUIDELINES

Initial phases of rehabilitation emphasize tissue healing, reduction of inflammation and pain, and protection of the repair. Immediately after surgery, patients are placed in an immobilizer, typically between 4 and 6 weeks. Pain and inflammation have been reported to inhibit shoulder musculature which is why the post-surgical team should make every effort to use cryotherapy and other modalities as necessary. Appropriate range of motion after surgery is important in order to minimize chances of developing post-operative stiffness.

As range of motion is achieved, proper exercise progression should be followed in order to limit stress on the healing repair. Throughout this process, healing of the rotator cuff repair should be respected.

The healing process is divided into three stages: inflammation (0–7 days), repair (5–14 days), and remodeling (> 14 days). One primate study showed an almost mature tendon-to-bone healing by 15 weeks after surgery. By 8 weeks, initiation of collagen alignment and organization was noticed. Sharpey fibers which hold the tendon and bone together did not appear in any considerable number until 12 weeks suggesting that excessive tension on the repair be avoided for 12 weeks post-surgery. Proposed rotator cuff repair guidelines (May be adjusted according to size of tear and quality of tissue)

Phase 1 (weeks 0–6)
- ROM

- FF to tolerance
- ER to 60° with arm in scapular plane
- IR: None

    - Weeks 0–2 weeks strict immobilization

- Distal hand and wrist activity

    - Squeezing, AROM hand and wrist
    - Weeks 2–4: continued immobilization

- PROM initiated by patient in scapular plane

    - 90° FF
    - 30° ER

- Continued hand and wrist exercises
- Elbow AROM with arm at side
- Scapular protraction/depression

    - Weeks 4–6: DC immobilizer

- PROM/AAROM with PT

    - Flexion, ER

- Supine PROM shoulder elevation

    - Criteria to advance

- Pain-free PROM
- FF beyond 120
- ER beyond 30

Phase 2 (weeks 7–11)
• ROM

- FF to tolerance
- ER to tolerance
- IR to beltline: no aggressive stretching

  • Week 7: progress AAROM ➜ AROM

- Supine Cane FF in scapular plane
- Incline cane FF ➜ standing cane
- Towel slide scaption
- Isometric exercise

  • ER/IR/Ext

- T band rows with retraction

  • Week 8:

- Standing shoulder extension

  • Criteria to advance

- Full, pain-free PROM
- Full AROM without compensation, no shoulder "shrug"
- Pain-free isometric exercises

Phase 3 (weeks 12+)
• ROM

- FF unrestricted
- ER unrestricted
- IR unrestricted

  • Week 12: strengthening

- T band ER/IR with towel

- Standing row
- Supine punch
- Side lying ER
- PNF diagonals
- Prone mid and low traps

Role of the scapula

The importance of the scapula is often underemphasized during rehabilitation of the shoulder. The scapula plays an essential role in shoulder function and stability of the glenohumeral joint. In patients with shoulder injuries, alterations in scapular position and motion have been reported 68–100% of the time. As the humerus is moving through space, it is important for the scapula to move as well to maintain centralization of the humeral head in the glenoid. The scapula has the capacity to move in three planes which include the ability to elevate/ depress, protract/retract, upward/downward rotation, internally/externally rotate, and tip anterior/ posterior around the thorax. Alterations in scapular position will commonly lead to shoulder dysfunction which is why all associated impairments must be addressed. Dysfunction of the scapula has been termed "scapular dyskinesis" and has been classified by Kibler as type I, II, and III; type I is identified as prominence of the inferior medial scapular border, type II, prominence of the medial scapular border and abnormal rotation, and type III, superior translation of the scapula and prominence of the superior medial border. In the early phases of post-operative rehab after rotator cuff repair, the patient can safely be placed in a side-lying position with the shoulder unweighted and perform scapular neuromuscular education activities with manual cues if needed. If this is started early in the post-surgical care, by the time rotator cuff specific exercises mcan be initiated, a sound scapular foundation has already been established.

Range of motion

During post-operative rehabilitation, it is important to protect the repair, promote tendon-to-bone healing, and minimize gapping between the tendon edges and its bony insertion. Early and immediate passive motion after surgery was once believed to help reduce post-operative stiffness; however, recent animal models suggest that this immediate motion can be detrimental. Immediate post-operative immobilization has been seen to result in better tendon–bone healing than immediate post-operative mobilization. Another animal model has shown that immediate early passive motion should be avoided and that delayed passive motion had no negative effect on the strength and maturity of the remodeled tendon. Early passive motion may stimulate excessive matrix formation and increased scar formation in the subacromial space which leads to worsening passive shoulder mechanics, increased stiffness, and loss of motion. A 2-week period of immobilization helps extracellular matrix represent similar characteristics of uninjured tissue. This period of immobilization results in increased type I collagen organization and less scar formation compared to early mobilization, concluding that the quality of tissue improves with decreased loads. These decreased loads on the tissue during early healing may provide a protective environment that allows for proper tendon-to-bone integration. As passive range of motion (ROM) is initiated after a 4–6-week period of immobilization, knowledge of strain on individual muscles and tendons can be beneficial. It is important to minimize activation and strain of the repaired tissue, which is why passive motion is performed first followed by active assisted and lastly active motion. After repair of the supraspinatus tendon, tensile strength of the rotator cuff significantly decreases when the arm is elevated more than 30° in the scapular plane. Strain significantly increases as the arm is lowered from 30° to 0° of elevation. Using a towel roll or support under the patients elbow when they are supine can help unload the repaired supraspinatus, and the patient should be educated to do the same at home when they are in the supine position to minimize strain. During passive elevation in the scapular plane, supraspinatus force remained near zero; however, forces were higher with the armplaced in the sagittal plane. The clinician should make every effort to provide ROM in the scapular plane to minimize stress. The scapular plane can easily be described as 30° from the midline. While advancing shoulder flexion, although strain decreases, redundancy in the soft tissue has potential to cause impingement or irritation in the subacromial space. As therapists progress into increased ranges of glenohumeral flexion, caution must be taken not to force beyond its point of first resistance and avoid end-range discomfort or pain. In the scapular plane, glenohumeral external rotation ranging from 0° to 60° constitutes a safe zone of motion which also puts minimal stress on a repaired supraspinatus. Increased external rotation beyond 60° has the potential to cause increased tension in the anterior portion of the tendon.

Significant increase in strain has been reported with internal rotation stretching after RC repair and therefore should be avoided.

Electromyographic (EMG) analysis of the supraspinatus confirms that therapist assisted shoulder elevation and external rotation, and pendulums performed by the patient are truly passive as these motions elicit activity similar to resting levels. However, EMG data reveals that with incorrectly performed pendulums moderate activity of the supraspinatus is generated and therefore may be avoided in early rehabilitation programs to minimize chance of patient error. When correctly performing pendulums, the patients position themselves slightly bent over, supported with their non-surgical arm. Shifting their bodyweight forward and backwards allows the arm to swing in a controlled manner with the assistance of gravity and not active muscle contraction. If pendulums are to be utilized, proper patient education and monitoring should be implemented to avoid unwanted activation of the rotator cuff. Although less common than supraspinatus, an injury to the subscapularis requires additional precautions. After a rotator cuff repair involving the subscapularis, precautions may change due to the portion of tendon that was repaired (superior vs. inferior). During forward flexion, there is minimal lengthening in the superior portion, whereas strain is increased on the inferior portion. With external rotation, there was increased strain on both portions of the tendon. Repair to the superior portion of this tendon would be favourable and a safe zone of forward flexion ranges from 0° to 90°. With repair to the inferior portion, forward flexion should be avoided in the early post-operative period to minimize stress on the repair. Also, any external rotation beyond neutral is contraindicated for this population.

Exercise progression

During strengthening of the rotator cuff, it is important that centralization of the humeral head is maintained and every attempt should be made to prevent superior migration. Superior migration of the humeral head, observed as a "shrug" during exercises can promote impingement of the healing tissue in the subacromial space. This "shrug" sign is also an indicator to the clinician that there is insufficient activation of the rotator cuff and altered mechanics within the glenohumeral joint. During strength progression, scapular positioning and muscle activation will be addressed since it is equally important in the recovery of this group of patients. Proper posture after surgery and sufficient muscle balance between scapular upward and downward rotators must be established. Scapular retraction and downward rotation can increase subacromial space and help promote a healing environment. During activity progression, patients are taken from passive to active assisted and finally active exercises in order to gradually load the repaired tissue in a slow and safe manner. EMG evidence suggests that forward bow exercise as well as supine PROM with the opposite hand all had very low levels of activity on the supraspinatus. Supine PROM by a therapist elicits very low and safe levels of supraspinatus and infraspinatus activity. During the forward bow exercise, the patients have their hand and forearm supported on a flat surface and step away from the hand allowing for passive shoulder elevation. Murphy also showed low EMG activity in both supraspinatus and infraspinatus in therapist assisted elevation, self- and therapist-assisted ER, and isometric IR. Whereas, pulleys, scapular retraction, and isometric ER all elicited EMG levels of supraspinatus and infraspinatus above baseline and are categorized as active exercises, not to be used in early rehab protocols. Once patients display minimal-to-no reported pain, acceptable passive ROM approaching 120° elevation in the scapular plane and tolerance of passive exercises without compensation, a transition to AAROM and upright activities can commence. When transitioning out of the gravity-eliminated position, exercises that place moderate stress on the rotator cuff tendons should be performed prior to high-stress activities. Safe active assistive exercises in this phase include supine wand flexion, progressed to incline wand flexion, and finally standing-assisted flexion along with ball rollout. Wall walk exercises elicited higher supraspinatus activation and should be used in late stages of AAROM prior to active forward elevation. Supported vertical wall slides generate less EMG activity and may be a better option than wall walks in the early stages. A preferred exercise of the author in this phase is a wall slide with a towel in the scapular plane which will promote co-contraction of the shoulder stabilizers while training shoulder elevation. As patients progress, wall slide with lift-off and eccentric lowering is initiated and finally active shoulder flexion in the scapular plane monitoring for a "shrug" sign throughout the available range of motion. The goals of intermediate phases of rehabilitation are to restore full ROM while adding basic and functional strengthening to combat immobilization and deconditioning. Selecting exercises that engage the rotator cuff as a coactivator rather than in isolation may benefit the patient while decreasing risks of complication. Isometric exercises performed in sub-maximal and sub-painful levels are initiated starting with internal and followed by external rotation.

During this time, scapular exercises are initiated as well. Standing-resisted shoulder extension and prone extension along with seated and prone row have all been shown to elicit high EMG levels of the targeted muscles without harmful strain on the supraspinatus.

During later stages of rehabilitation, advanced rotator cuff exercises are initiated. Following our healing principles that excessive strain prior to 12 weeks may be harmful, we can now progress exercise that load the supraspinatus. External rotation(ER) at 0° abduction with a towel has been reported to produce activation up to 41% of maximum voluntary isometric contraction (MVIC) and may be initiated. Side-lying resisted ER, diagonal exercises as well as prone horizontal abduction, and external rotation are all appropriate for this later stage.

As the rehabilitation program evolves, strengthening should become more targeted toward the rotator cuff. EMG studies comparing various positions for external rotation show highest activation of supraspinatus during ER performed at 90° abduction in the cocking position, suggesting this exercise may best be implemented toward the later stages of rehabilitation. Additionally, prone ER in 90° abduction followed by side lying ER with resistance showed highest activation of the infraspinatus. Conversely, IR performed in 90° abduction has been shown to have higher activation of supraspinatus, infraspinatus, and subscapularis when compared to IR at side. As expected, when moving into a more advanced and sport-specific position required for overhead athletes, the demands of the rotator cuff increase as does its activation. These exercises should be reserved for end stage rehab for athletes and may not be ideal for those who do not need to return to a throwing sport. Although they have the highest MVIC for the rotator cuff showing best isolation, they are also performed at end range and in a position that may provoke impingement should the patient not have the appropriate motion or control. While rotational strength is important in post-operative rehab, it is also important to consider the contractile tissue involved in scapular stability. These muscles help control dynamic scapular motion; provide force couples, and a foundation for the shoulder joint. Most noted in the research is the concept that over activation of the upper trapezius and under activation of the middle and lower trapezius promotes poor scapular position and shoulder impingement. Impairment of the serratus anterior also causes altered scapular kinematics and will also promote shoulder impingement if not addressed. Ideal exercises in shoulder rehab enhance activation of the above mentioned muscles with minimal input from the upper traps. High serratus anterior activation has been reported with supine punch performed at 90°

and 120°. Hardwick et al. showed the wall slide to be an effective exercise to engage the serratus anterior at elevation angles of 90° and above. The wall slide was performed with the ulnar borders of both arms in contact with the wall at 90° of elevation. The shoulders were elevated in a plane approximating the scapular plane. The subjects were instructed to slide the forearms up the wall, while leaning into it by transferring body weight from the non-dominant foot to the dominant foot. High middle trap activity occurs with prone rowing and prone horizontal abduction at 90°. Greatest lower trap EMG activity has been reported in prone full can, prone ER at 90° abduction, bilateral external rotation, and prone horizontal abduction at 90° with ER. Side-lying ER has also been shown to have high levels of lower trap activity, which may be useful as it also has high activity of the posterior rotator cuff.

The rhomboids play a role as scapular retractors and depressors and are engaged during most of the abovementioned exercises. In addition to the above exercises, prone extension and prone row have high EMG activity of the rhomboids and should be included in shoulder strengthening programs.

CONCLUSION

Rehabilitation after rotator cuff repair must follow criteria based progression taking into account healing of the repaired tissue. With a firm understanding of the anatomy, healing properties, strain, and tissue loading, programs can be individualized to each patient. It is imperative for the patient to understand these guiding principles as well so that realistic expectations can be established and desired outcomes can be achieved in a timely manner.

CHAPTER FIVE

CUBITAL TUNNEL SYNDROME

INTRODUCTION

Although the incidence of cubital tunnel has not been well reported, it is estimated to be around 1% in United States. Ulnar nerve compression is the second most common nerve entrapment of the upper extremity after carpal tunnel syndrome. Ulnar nerve can be entrapped at multiple sites of the upper extremity, from the cervical nerve roots C8/T1 and brachial plexus to more distal sites at the elbow, forearm and wrist. Elbow entrapment is seen most commonly and has been referred to as the tardy ulnar nerve palsy in the past. 'Cubital tunnel syndrome' is the term introduced by Feindel and Stratford in 1958 because of its similarity to carpal tunnel syndrome.

PATHOLOGY OF NERVE COMPRESSION

Anatomical factors

Multiple sites of compression of the ulnar nerve have been identified around the elbow. The most proximal site of compression around the elbow involves the arcade of Struthers. The arcade of Struthers is a hiatus in the medial intermuscular septum approximately 8cm proximal to the medial epicondyle. This thickening of deep fascia of distal arm that extends between medial head of the triceps and the intermuscular septum is present in 70% of people. Another reported site of compression is the medial intermuscular septum itself. Osborne was the first to describe another more distal site of compression. This transverse band crosses the ulnar nerve just distal to the medial epicondyle and is termed Osborne's ligament. It is the most commonly identified site of compression of the ulnar nerve at the elbow. Additionally, a thick facial band between the two heads of flexor carpi ulnaris has also been implicated in some cases. Appreciation of the multiple sites of compression is crucial, so that each site can be evaluated during surgery for successful release Space occupying lesions Multiple pathological conditions that occupy the cubital tunnel can cause cubital tunnel syndrome. Those lesions include tumors, ganglions, bony spurs, medial epicondyle nonunions from previous fractures, hypertrophic callus, synovitis in rheumatoid arthritis or gout, as well as hematoma formation in hemophiliacs or patients on blood thinners. In most cases of cubital tunnel syndrome no space occupying lesion can be identified.

Intrinsic stretch

Given that symptoms of cubital tunnel syndrome are exacerbated with elbow flexion, there has been much debate about relative importance of external compression versus intrinsic traction. Previous studies that used pressure measurements in the cubital tunnel showed both types of mechanisms at work, but they were not able to show the amount of contribution from each mechanism specifically. More recently, Gelberman et al looked at both the interstitial and extraneural pressures on the ulnar nerve at the cubital tunnel using pressure measuring catheters as well as MRI to evaluate compression and

cubital tunnel volume change with elbow flexion. They noticed much larger increase in intraneural pressure compared to extraneural pressure with no evidence of direct compression. This data points to traction of the ulnar nerve with elbow flexion to be more likely the major contributor to increased intraneural pressure and symptomology. This information would incline the surgeon to transpose the nerve, instead of releasing the compression alone.

CLINICAL FEATURES

Patients with cubital tunnel syndrome present with paresthesias over the small and ring fingers. Paresthesias present early in the disease and progress to motor dysfunction as the compression of the nerve becomes more severe and chronic. Intrinsic muscle weakness, as well as, weakness of flexor digitorum profoundus of small and ring fingers can be seen in more advanced disease, which presents as clawing. Sparing of flexor digitorum profoundus (FDP) is seen with more distal compression, such as seen at Guyon's canal and can help with differential diagnosis. This FDP sparing is called ulnar paradox, which means that the more distal the lesion is on the ulnar nerve the less clawing is noted due to decreased involvement of flexor digitorum profoundus with more distal lesions. Patient also can complain of their small finger getting caught when trying to place their hand in a pocket of their pants. This is due to overpower of small finger extensor without opposition of interosseous muscles causing small finger abduction and is called Wartenberg sign.

On physical exam there is a positive tinel sign over the cubital tunnel. Froment sign is noted due to weakness of adductor pollicis muscle. Froment sign is positive when a patient is given a piece of paper and holds it together between the thumb and index finger with flexion of the thumb IP joint. Positive flexion sign at the elbow with supination and wrist extension reproducing the symptoms up to 60 seconds and ulnar nerve subluxation with elbow flexion can also be seen. Still, flexion and tinel signs have been noted to be falsely positive in up to 24% of cases. False positive results could also be due to the fact that, even under normal elbow flexion conduction velocity and intraneural pressure can decrease as described previously in cadaveric studies. Tenderness over the hook of hamate or pisiform should be evaluated to rule out compression at the guyon's canal. Abnormal finger flexion and loss of dorsal sensory branch of the ulnar nerve as seen in cubital tunnel compression can help in differentiating it from Guyon's canal pathology. Spurling test should be used to check for cervical causes of symptoms. Hand diagram for patient is often used to help portray the involvement of the sensory ulnar nerve distribution to the examiner.

Many diagnostic studies are helpful in confirming the suspected diagnosis and can also rule out specific causes of cubital tunnel compression. Plain X-rays should be obtained to look for degenerative changes of the cervical spine and elbow, as well as bony compression from spurs or previous fractures. Neurophysiological studies are helpful in establishing diagnosis and should be done if surgery is planned, in order to document preoperative baseline. Ulnar nerve velocity of <50 m/s at the elbow I considered positive for cubital tunnel syndrome.

TREATMENT AND OUTCOMES

Conservative, nonsurgical treatments should be tried initially as they are effective in relieve of the symptoms in up to 50% of the cases. Nonsurgical treatment should be tried for at least 3 months before surgical intervention, especially in mild cases. NSAIDs, activity modification that eliminates prolonged elbow flexion as well as nighttime splinting at 45 degrees of flexion and the use of elbow pad, have been described with good results. Vitamin B6 use is controversial and there is no concrete data to support its use. Most of the evidence for vitamin B6 stems from treatment of carpal tunnel syndrome.

There are three commonly used surgical treatments and there are proponents for use of each treatment. First type of surgical treatment is simple decompression, by either open or endoscopic release of the Osborne's band. This is reserved for mild cases, with recent onset of symptoms and mild sensory changes on the nerve studies. Advantages include simple operation, less devascularization of the nerve and less scarring. Disadvantages include limited decompression and possibly missing compression at other sites. Endoscopic decompression has also been described in the literature. In a recent study by Bultmann, 47 patients with various levels of severity of cubital tunnel syndrome underwent endoscopic release with 98% reporting good to excellent results after the surgery. Majority of those patients did not have strength loss preoperatively suggesting milder cubital tunnel syndrome, but their sensation has improved to normal levels in 94% of cases. Other studies have described good results in about 78% of the patients. Endoscopic decompression can have similar indications as simple decompression. The second type of surgical treatment which involves medial epicondylectomy has also been used to relieve cubital tunnel syndrome, especially with visible compression from osteophytes and previous fractures of distal humerus. Advantages include specific and more extensive decompression, but there is higher risk of causing nerve subluxation, which can lead to continued symptoms.

Goldberg et al. retrospectively analyzed 48 medial epicondylectomy procedures in 46 patients and noted improvement of symptoms in 98% of the patients, although strength improved only in about half of the patients. Worse results were seen with more severe preoperative function. Third surgical technique is anterior transposition of the ulnar nerve with placement of the nerve subcutaneous, submuscular or intramuscular. Advantages include thorough release of ulnar nerve and evaluation of multiple sites of compression. Theoretical disadvantages include decrease blood supply to the nerve from soft tissue dissection, as well as higher likelihood of nerve injury from manipulation and complexity of the procedure.

A recent meta-analysis by Macadam et al based on 10 studies showed no statistically significant difference between simple decompression and nerve transposistion but only a trend toward improved results with transposition of the ulnar nerve. Dr. Kevin Chung did another mataanalysis of previous studies. Those studies included extensive review by Bartels et al. who analyzed studies between 1970 and 1997 and noted that if patients were not evaluated base on severity of symptoms, simple decompression had better results. On the other hand, when controlled for severity results were very similar. Another study by Mowlavi et al. which analyzed 30 published studies from 1945 to 1995 showed good surgical outcomes for mild to moderate disease and poor outcomes for severe disease with any types of surgical procedures. Limitations of previous studies included low power and poor data quality. Dr. Chung came to conclusion that given no clear evidence of better results with extensile procedures, simple decompression should be favored as the initial surgical procedure. A study by Adelaar et al., showed similar results for simple versus subcutaneous and submuscular release with all severity of cubital tunnel syndromes grouped together, but slightly better results with moderate degree of compression when using submuscular transposition. Submuscular transposition

has also been commonly used for recurrent cubital tunnel syndrome, but recent studies have showed good results with subcutaneous transposition as well.

A recent study by Keiner et al., looked at 33 patient treated with either submuscular transposition or simple decompression over longer follow up of at least 3 years. 10 of 16 patient in transposition group and 11 of 17 patients in decompression group were completely free of symptoms. Although study sample was small, no difference was found between the two groups' long term and authors recommended simple decompression as a less invasive procedure.

Again, review of multiple studies fails to show one superior procedure with improved outcomes when comparing between different types of decompressions. This is especially true for mild to moderate forms of cubital tunnel syndrome. In those cases simple decompression is often chosen due to minimally invasive nature of this approach. In other patient with severe stage of the disease, cubitus valgus and nerve sublaxation, anterior transposition procedures should be strongly considered. Further randomized prospective, multicenter studies are needed to improve power of the results. Further future studies should include a more specific pre operative evaluation of severity of the disease and post surgical evaluation of outcomes.

The author prefers using subcutaneous transposition of the ulnar nerve paying attention to the inferior ulnar collateral artery as the main supply to the transposed nerve. Technique involves making a 10 cm incision posterior to the medial epicondyle, with the epicondyle being in the center of the incision. Inferior ulnar collateral vessles are about 2.5 cm proximal to the medial epicondyle. During the dissection to the ulnar nerve, care is taken to protect the medial antebrachial cutanious nerve to the forearm. Ulnar nerve is then dissected out insitu. Attention is then directed at isolating and protecting the ulnar collateral artery supplying the nerve. This is done by careful elevation and resection of the medial intermuscular septum around the vessel. After protection of the vessel and the mesoneurium, the nerve is transposed anteriorly and freed at all proximal and distal compression sites mentioned before. A single fascial flap 1 × 2 cm in size is then created from the fascia of the common flexor mass to secure the nerve at a subcutaneous anterior location. This flap is sutures loosely to allow for unobstructed gliding of lateralized nerve after transposition. Finally, the nerve is checked for smooth gliding and no other sites of compression at its new location with full range of motion of the elbow. Patient is then splinted and started on early range of motion of the elbow to prevent elbow stiffness and scar formation.

Complications and failure

Posterior branch of the medial antebrachial cutaneous nerve is a common complication especially during endoscopic procedures. This injury can present as painful scar or hyperesthesia in the medial forearm. Persistent symptoms of cubital tunnel syndrome are often present due to incomplete release of the ulnar nerve or postoperative scarring. Early motion of the elbow can help prevent adhesions, which are more likely to occur with sub- muscular transpositions because of muscle detachment. Subluxation of ulnar nerve can occur with simple decompression or medial epicondylectomy, leading to persistent symptoms. Thus, after simple decompression or medial epicondylectomy, the surgeon should check for ulnar nerve subluxation and convert the procedure to transposition to secure the ulnar nerve if subluxation is noted. Medial collateral ligament can also be injured with more extensive submuscular decompression or medial epicondylectomy.

CONCLUSION

Cubital tunnel syndrome is common but not fully understood. Multiple sites of compression of the ulnar nerve at the elbow make it difficult to treat cases that are resistant to the mainstay therapy. It is thus crucial to correlate both the history and physical exam to provide the best type of procedure for each patient limiting the risk of complications. Fortunately, most cases of ulnar nerve compression improve with nonsurgical treatment and large majority get better with surgical decompression. The fact that most people get better with and without surgical treatment is likely the reason that multiple studies have failed to show improved results with different types of decompressions for mild cubital tunnel syndrome. Transposition surgeries have been shown to yield better results with more severe cases and patients who failed previous simple releases, likely secondary to release of other compression sites that were missed by the initial surgery. For mild to moderate cases of cubital tunnel simple decompression might be the procedure of choice due to its lower complexity and lack of evidence of worse results compared to other decompressive procedures. Knowing more about pathology of the cutbital tunnel syndrome such as compression versus traction injury and having better modalities for evaluation of the nerve should help us to better tailor treatment for the patients in the future.

CHAPTER SIX

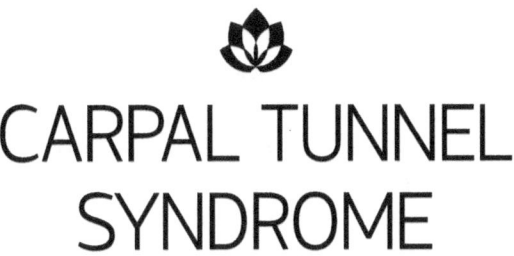

CARPAL TUNNEL SYNDROME

INTRODUCTION
Carpal tunnel syndrome (CTS) is the commonest peripheral nerve problem in the United Kingdom and has considerable employment and healthcare costs. If recognised early it is readily treatable. No established UK guidelines exist for diagnosis and management, but the American Academy of Neurology issued guidelines in 1993, which remain current as no major recent advances have occurred.

ETIOLOGY
Carpal tunnel syndrome results from compromise of median nerve function at the wrist caused by increased pressure in the carpal tunnel, an anatomical compartment bounded by the bones of the carpus and the transverse carpal ligament. Although the ends of the tunnel are in free communication with the surrounding tissues, tissue pressure in the tunnel is much higher in patients with CTS (32-110mmHg, depending on wrist position) than in patients with normal wrists (2-31 mm Hg.2 Pressures are raised by wrist flexion and extension, and finger flexion. Intermittent or sustained high tissue pressure in the tunnel impairs microvascular circulation in the median nerve and leads to spurious generation of action potentials, local demyelination, and ultimately axonal loss. It may also stimulate the proliferation of subsynovial connective tissue in the tunnel, according to pathological studies of CTS.

Anything that reduces the dimensions of the tunnel or increases the volume of its contents will predispose to CTS, and many medical associations have been reported, but most cases are idiopathic. A study of 4488 individuals recruited from the St Thomas' UK adult twin registry found genetic predisposition to be the single strongest factor in predicting the development of the syndrome. Obesity is a risk factor in younger patients. The role of occupational and recreational hand use in causation remains controversial. If overuse of the hands does contribute, it may be a relatively minor factor, though most patients report that heavy use of the hands aggravates the symptoms. A Scandinavian survey found population prevalences of 14.4% for median nerve distribution paraesthesias, 3.8% for CTS diagnosed on clinical grounds, 4.9% for neurophysiological focal impairment of the median nerve at the wrist, and 2.7% for neurophysiologically confirmed clinical CTS.

Incidence peaks in the late 50s, particularly in women, and the late 70s, when the sex ratio is more equal. It is also common, transiently, in late pregnancy. Elderly people tend to present with more severe CTS for the same length of history, with 59% of patients aged over 65 having thenar atrophy at presentation comparedwith 18% of younger patients.8 CTS in older patients is easily confused with other, less treatable, disorders.

Although the syndrome encompasses a range of severity (from transient subjective sensory symptoms to irreversible thenar wasting and sensory loss) it should be recognised before permanent deficits develop. Patients woken by paraesthesias or pain—the distribution of which includes median nerve territory (the thumb and first two and a half fingers)—have CTS until proved otherwise.

Some patients will also complain of sensory disturbance in the whole hand or pain radiating up the arm to the shoulder. Patients whose paraesthesias are limited to the ulnar side of the hand are unlikely to have CTS.

About 55%-65% of cases are bilateral at first presentation and most patients present first with the dominant hand. Daytime symptoms may be noticed with particular activities, particularly those that involve holding the arms raised. Patients may complain of a perception of swelling of the hand or fingers, but visible swelling is rare and should prompt consideration of other conditions with secondary CTS. Sensory loss in median nerve territory and weakness and wasting of the median innervated thenar muscles are reliable but late indicators of CTS.

The American Academy of Neurology's guidelines state that the likelihood of a diagnosis increases with the number of standard symptoms and provocative factors present. The most widely used provocative physical tests are Phalen's sign (the provocation of median paraesthesias by flexion of the wrist to 90o for 60 seconds) and Tinel's sign (the provocation of paraesthesias by tapping over the carpal tunnel).

SYMPTOMS
- Dull, aching discomfort in the hand, forearm, or upper arm
- Paraesthesias in the hand
- Weakness or clumsiness of the hand
- Dry skin, swelling, or colour changes in the hand
- Occurrence of any of the above in the median distribution
- Provocation of symptoms by sleep
- Provocation of symptoms by sustained hand or arm positions
- Provocation of symptoms by repetitive actions of the hand or wrist
- Mitigation of symptoms by changing hand posture or shaking the wrist

*According to the American Academy of Neurology's guideline

These signs have been compared with nerve conduction studies as a diagnostic gold standard in many studies. In such studies, Phalen's sign has sensitivity ranging from 10% to 73% and specificity from 55% to 86%. Tinel's sign has sensitivity ranging from 8% to 100% and specificity from 55% to 87%, the wide ranges probably reflecting the difficulty in standardising the test methods. Both signs are less reliable in advanced CTS. On general examination of the patient, be alert for signs of endocrine disease and connective tissue disorders, which can predispose to CTS, and other hand problems such as Raynaud's phenomenon, vibration white finger, trigger finger, and Dupuytren's contracture, which can all coexist with CTS.

INVESTIGATIONS

Plain x ray examination of the hand is not cost effective in idiopathic CTS—an American study concluded that costs were $5869 (£2850; €4250) to $20 115 for each finding of therapeutic significance.

A check for diabetes, however, is inexpensive and appropriate. Most patients with CTS will be in an age group where undetected hyperglycaemia is common. The value of blood tests to screen for connective tissue disease and thyroid function is uncertain, particularly in the absence of any clinical indication other than CTS.

Complex investigations are not necessary before starting conservative treatment in clinically obvious cases. However, in cases of diagnostic doubt, and before surgery, nerve conduction studies should be carried out.

The American Academy of Neurology's guidelines suggest electrodiagnostic studies and therapeutic trials with non-invasive treatment as the strategies of choice when clinical diagnosis is uncertain. Nerve conduction studies should include sufficient measurements to localise median nerve dysfunction to the carpal tunnel, evaluate its severity, and exclude more widespread neuropathy.

Neurophysiological severity of CTS can be expressed on the 7 points

Canterbury scale (0=no abnormality, 6=no recordable median motor or sensory potentials), which have shown correlates with surgical prognosis.

However, nerve conduction studies have a small false negative rate; a precise figure is not available for this because no better test exists for comparison as a gold standard. However, with modern nerve conduction studies, it is probably around 5-10%. In east Kent, 4.3% of 3544 successful carpal tunnel decompressions had normal preoperative nerve conduction studies (unpublished personal data). Conversely not all patients with a neurophysiologically demonstrated median neuropathy at the wrist necessarily have symptoms related to that.

An alternative, or ideally complementary, approach is provided by high resolution ultrasonography of the median nerve. In a blind comparison with nerve conduction studies as a gold standard, ultrasonography achieved 89% sensitivity and 69% specificity. However, this study retrospectively optimised the ultrasound measurement cut-off values to achieve the best possible diagnostic performance and is limited in any case by the lack of an absolute diagnostic standard for comparison.

Magnetic resonance imaging can make similar measurements of median nerve dimensions but is more expensive. Ultrasonography is more comfortable than nerve conduction studies for patients but will not detect other nerve problems that may be contributing to the presentation. Ultrasonography may show unsuspected structural abnormalities of relevance, such as bifid median nerves, persistent median arteries, or space occupying lesions in the tunnel, but these are rare and even more rarely do they dictate alternative management.

DIFFERENTIAL DIAGNOSIS

• Cervical radiculopathy (especially C6/7)—look for local neck pain on movement and neurological signs outside the territory of the distal median nerve.

• Ulnar neuropathy—this can also produce nocturnal paraesthesias; the distribution will usually be to the medial side of the hand.

• Raynaud's phenomenon—this should be recognisable from a history of symptoms related to cold exposure.

- Vibration white finger—suspect this if the patient uses vibrating hand tools at work.
- Osteoarthritis of the metacarpophalangeal joint of the thumb—this can produce a spurious appearance of thenar wasting but not true weakness or sensory deficit.
- Tendonitis—specific tests may help in diagnosis, such as Finkelstein's test for De Quervain's tenosynovitis.
- Generalised peripheral neuropathies—these should be recognised from the wider distribution of symptoms and reflex changes.
- Motor neurone disease—this can present with wasting in one hand but does not produce sensory symptoms.
- Syringomyelia—features such as prominent loss of temperature sensation in the hands should give a clue.
- Multiple sclerosis—this should be recognised from the presence of neurological abnormalities disseminated in location and time.

TREATMENT

Many treatments, both conventional and complementary, have been suggested for CTS. Few are supported by good quality evidence from randomised controlled trials.

The recommendations of the American Academy of Neurology for treatment remain reasonable. The academy suggests splinting, activity modification, and non-steroidal anti-inflammatory drugs—and possibly diuretics if there is limb swelling—as conservative treatment, followed by steroid injection and surgery if these fail or in patients with progressive motor deficit.

However, activity modification, diuretics, and nonsteroidal anti-inflammatory drugs have no positive support from any randomised trials. Meta-analysis of several randomised trials shows that vitamin B-6 supplementation has a negligible therapeutic effect. The purpose of treatment is to alleviate the symptoms and, in some people, prevent worsening of the condition.

A few, mostly elderly, patients have thenar wasting but no symptoms. Little is to be gained from surgery in such cases.

CTS is not necessarily progressive. The condition in some patients may fluctuate slightly for many years— with more symptoms during periods of heavy hand use or variation with the seasons—without progressing to irreversible median nerve damage. The condition may even remit spontaneously. In one study 23% of participants improved over 12-15 months without active intervention though this was not a randomised trial and the researchers were not able to rigorously control factors such as activity modification instituted by the patients. The potential benefits of treatment must be viewed against this background.

Splinting

A removable wrist brace that maintains the wrist at a neutral angle without applying direct compression over the carpal tunnel provides mechanical respite for the nerve. Such supports are often too cumbersome for daytime use, but for those patients who tolerate them at night, they are often an effective way of achieving an undisturbed night's sleep. In a trial comparing splinting with surgery,37%of patients in the splint group obtained satisfactory symptom relief from this measure alone, and splints have the advantage of being inexpensive (£3.50 each) and without serious adverse effects.

Steroids

Carpal tunnel syndrome has been shown to respond to both systemic steroids and to local steroids given at (or near) the wrist by either injection or iontophoresis (transdermal delivery driven by an electric field). The side effects of oral steroids preclude their routine use for CTS, but local steroid injection has no discernible systemic effects and a very low incidence of local complications. Although median nerve damage from intraneural injection has been reported in eight cases, pooling the reported trials of steroid injection yields a total of over 3000 injections performed without serious complications, and the risk may be estimated at <0.1% in competent hands. The initial response rate to a single steroid injection is about 70%, but relapse is common. No adequate long term studies exist to allow precise quantification of the relapse rate beyond the first few months. The most pessimistic estimates suggest that 92% may have relapsed by two years. At the other extreme is a series in which half of injected patients remain in remission at seven years. No evidence is available to guide policy on treatment after relapse following a successful first injection, though it is common practice to inject a second or sometimes third time, and there are anecdotal reports of patients maintained long term on repeated injections.

Surgery

Carpal tunnel decompression, usually performed as a day case under local anaesthesia, is considered the definitive treatment. However, although it provides permanent and complete cure in most cases, it is not without risk. A survey of over 4000 patients having surgery under usual NHS circumstances found that about two years after surgery, only 75% considered the operation an unqualified success and 8% thought that they were worse off. Although papers in the literature devoted to "recurrent CTS" are numerous, true recurrence, after successful initial surgery, is rare. It may be more common after endoscopic surgery.

Most reports in fact relate to primary failure of the operation to relieve symptoms. Such failures are mostly attributable to misdiagnosis (the symptoms actually being due to other causes, whether or not there is a median lesion at the wrist), surgical errors (the commonest being failure to fully divide the transverse carpal ligament), and delay of treatment to a point when median nerve function is beyond recovery.

A small minority are the result of more unpredictable surgical complications, inadvertent nerve and vessel lacerations, infections, painful scarring, and complex regional pain syndrome.

Although endoscopic methods of carpal tunnel decompression have been popular in recent years, long term outcomes do not differ significantly between the traditional and endoscopic approaches, and even the possible advantage of an earlier return to use of the hand after endoscopic surgery seems limited to a few days only. Despite the greater technical difficulty of endoscopic surgery, it does not seem to be associated with greater incidence of serious complications.

However, most published series of endoscopic procedures have been performed by enthusiasts for the technique who have achieved considerable technical proficiency. Some caution should therefore be shown before the widespread adoption of these methods by the occasional carpal tunnel surgeon.

Patients with CTS having surgery before reaching grade 6 on the Canterbury scale whose symptoms do not respond to surgery should have repeat nerve conduction studies performed within three months, and if these show no change or deterioration, re-exploration should be performed, particularly looking for incomplete ligament section.

Imaging studies may also be able to show this surgical mistake, but this has not yet been systematically reported. Overall, patients whose CTS symptoms are significantly troublesome and who have mild or moderate impairment of median nerve function should be offered splinting and local steroid injection.

Patients failing such conservative management and those who present at a later stage with objective neurological signs or delayed motor conduction on nerve conduction systems should be offered the option of surgical decompression. All should be advised of the potential risks of the different treatments.

Surgical decompression—open (several variations, with or without tenosynovectomy, transverse carpal ligament reconstruction, and external/internal neurolysis; all seem equally effective with no clear evidence to support the use of the more elaborate procedures); endoscopic (one or two portal).

Other treatments
- Diuretics
- Non-steroidal anti-inflammatory drugs
- Rest or activity modification
- Nerve and tendon gliding exercises
- Vitamin B-6
- Synovectomy only
- Chiropractic manipulation of the wrist
- Yoga
- Ultrasonography
- Acupuncture
- Serratiopeptidase
- Magnet therapy
- Cognitive behaviour therapy
- Lidoderm patches

CHAPTER SEVEN

ROTATOR CUFF CALCIFIC TENDINITIS

INTRODUCTION

Calcium deposit within the rotator cuff tendon is a common shoulder disorder. Calcium deposits may be in the form of calcific tendinitis or dystrophic calcification. Calcific tendinitis is calcification within a viable and well vascularized rotator cuff. It occurs within the midsubstance of the cuff, 1 to 2 cm proximal to its insertion. Classically, the condition will end by spontaneous resolution and it is uncommon to see other signs of degenerative changes.

Dystrophic calcification is calcification within a nonviable and poorly vascularized rotator cuff. It occurs at the insertion site or at the edges of a cuff tear. Classically, the condition worsens by time and it is common to see other signs of degenerative changes.

PREVALANCE

Calcific tendinitis usually occurs during the fifth and sixth decades of life. It occurs within the supraspinatus tendon in almost 50% of cases. It is more common in females (60%). It occurs more commonly with sedentary workers than with heavy labor workers (45% are house wives).

PATHOGENESIS AND NATURAL HISTORY

Controversy exists over the exact cause of calcific tendinitis. Burkhead and Gohlke proposed that it is a degenerative process that involves necrotic changes of tendon fibers that progress into dystrophic calcification. Mclaughlin believed that it proceeded from focal hyalinization of the fibers that become fibrillated and detached from the tendon, thus wounding up into rice-like bodies that later undergo calcification.

On the other hand, Uhthoff pointed out that this may be true regarding dystrophic calcification. But regarding calcific tendinitis they believed that this explanation was most unlikely. They argued that calcific tendinitis occurred in viable and well vascularised tissues and thus could not be a degenerative process; instead they suggested that it was a reparative process progressing through a predictable disease cycle. The calcium deposits may have a chalk-like consistency or a fluid consistency or a mixed one.

CLASSIFICATION

Many classifications have been suggested to describe calcific tendinitis. Some classified it according to the severity of the symptoms into acute, subacute and chronic.

Others classified it according to the radiological form into two categories. The first with localized, discrete, dense and homogenous deposits with spontaneous healing tendency and the second with diffuse, fluffy and heterogeneous deposits characterized by delayed and slow healing.

The French society of arthroscopy divided the condition into four types: Type A (20%) with homogenous deposits with well defined edges; Type B (45%) with heterogeneous fragmented deposits with well defined edges; Type C (30%) with heterogeneous deposits with ill defined edges and Type D which is not calcific tendinitis but degenerative dystrophic calcifications at the rotator cuff insertion.

Uhthoff *et al.* were the ones who described the complete cycle of the calcium deposits and explained the development of its natural history. They divided the condition into formative and resorptive phases. Lying within the two phases most authors motioned the presence of three stages; pre-calcification (silent), calcification (impingement) and post-calcification (acute). The chronic formative phase results from transient hypoxia that is commonly associated with repeated microtrauma and sometimes with a significant single trauma. This results in increased proteoglycan levels that induce tenocyte metaplasia into chondrocytes. This is followed by calcium deposits, mainly into the matrix vesicles within the chondrocytes. These deposits develop into bone foci that later coalesce. During the acute resorptive phase the periphery of the calcium deposits shows vascularization with macrophage and mononuclear giant cell infiltration together with fibroblast formation. This produces an aggressive inflammatory reaction with inflammatory cell accumulation, excessive edema and rise of the intratendineous pressure. This leads to severe pain which is attributed by some to secondary impingement resulting from the increased tendon size, or due to rupture of the deposits into the subacromial space or into the bursa. During the post-calcification stage the fibroblasts lay down collagen (mainly type II) that fills the gap. This will maturate into collagen type I within 12 to 16 months.

CLINICAL PRESENTATION

The clinical presentation is highly variable and depends on the phase the patient is passing through. During the chronic formative phase that may extend anywhere from 1 to 6 years, the patient may be completely asymptomatic. In some cases the condition will only be discovered accidentally. Some patients may present with symptoms that mimic mild impingement.

However during the acute resorptive phase, the patient usually presents with severe symptoms that may extend from 3 wk up to 6 months. In general, the more severe the symptoms are, the shorter the duration of the condition is. The patient presents with tremendous pain all over the shoulder with tenderness over the supraspinatus insertion. Pain commonly extends to the root of the neck with difficulty during overhead activity associated with muscle spasm. It is very difficult to perform any of the special tests due to the unbearable pain.

IMAGING

Radiological investigations confirm the diagnosis and may even make the diagnosis in asymptomatic cases. It also suggests the phase of the condition and is used to follow its progression.

They include conventional X-ray in true anteroposterior, lateral and outlet views. Deposits within the subscapularis may be detected by anteroposterior view in external rotation. In internal rotation, the deposits within the infraspinatus and teres minor may be detected. "Skullcap appearance" indicates rupture of the deposits within the bursa.

Ultrasonographic examination was reported to be more sensitive in detecting the calcium deposits within the cuff.

Computed tomography allowed better localization of the deposits. Although routine conventional X-ray allowed detection of the deposits, magnetic resonance imaging (MRI) studies allow better evaluation of any coexisting pathology. The deposits present with a low intensity signal in the T1 weighted images. In the T2 weighted images there may be perifocal low intensity signal denoting surrounding edema. The thinned out cuff lateral to the deposits may be falsely interpreted as a cuff tear. MRI arthrography was more beneficial to avoid such false conclusions.

TREATMENT

Various methods of treatment have been suggested. The appropriate method should be individualized for each patient depending on proper understanding of the pathophysiology and natural history of the condition, as well as proper clinical and radiological assessment of the patient, and finally accurate determination of the stage at which the patient presents. The treatment may be "conservative" including pain killers and physiotherapy, or "minimally invasive" as needling and puncture and aspiration or "operative" whether arthroscopic or open.

Due to the intolerable pain of the acute and severely painful resorptive stage, the patient often demands any sort of intervention despite explaining to him that the condition is probably resolving. Since the natural history of the condition ends with resorption of the deposits and complete relief of pain, usually conservative measures are successful in most of cases, reaching 80% in some studies and even 99% in others.

During the acute stage the aim is to relief of pain. The efficacy of non-steroidal drugs may be doubtful with frequent need to narcotic medications.

Physiotherapy

Some authors suggested physiotherapy including range of motion exercises to avoid gleno-humeral stiffness and idiopathic frozen shoulder. However there is no evidence that calcific tendinitis causes gleno-humeral capsular contracture. There is no solid evidence that different physical modalities including infrared, ultrasound, or deep heat have any effect on the natural history of the condition.

Extracorporeal shock wave

Extracorporeal shock wave (ECSW) has been used to treat symptomatic patients passing through the chronic formative phase with definite radiological evidence of calcium deposits. Most authors report short term symptomatic improvement. But ECSW was not free from complications, that included transient bone marrow edema and even reported cases of humeral head necrosis.

Most authors reported that the improvement is dose dependant, with better results following one or two sessions of high energy applications.

Needling or puncture and lavage

Minimally invasive techniques include needling or puncture and aspiration. These techniques were suggested by many authors aiming at decompressing the deposits and thus relieving the pain. They suggested that direct puncture of the deposits would shorten the natural history of the condition and accelerate resorption in 50% of cases.

Since the fifties of the last century some authors recommended blind needling of the deposits with intralesional local anesthetic injection reporting pain relief in 85% of cases. They reported that the amount of deposits removed didn't affect the outcome and accordingly concluded that pierce opening of the deposits was the essential step and not the calcium removal.

In the sixties Depalma and Kruper popularized blind needling of the deposits without any radiological localization, with good results. Clement reported pain relief within 24 hr following repeated blind needling of the deposits (15 to 20 times), after local anesthetic and corticosteroid injection into the subacromial space. He referred the patients to ultrasonic treatment within a few days. He claimed that this would cause active hyperemia that would enhance deposit absorption.

Most authors reported very good results after performing needling under fluoroscopic and, or ultrasonographic guidance. Local corticosteroid injection (whether intralesional or into the subacromial space) following the needling of the deposits, is recommended by some authors with good results and some suggested two or more injections.

Many studies showed no evidence that corticosteroid injection improved the results. Some reported that corticosteroids injection was short acting and only symptomatic. Other surgeons argued that corticosteroids would reduce the tendon healing process. Neer disagreed with this claim.

Many authors recommended dual needling and lavage for cases with calcium deposits. Needling is no new technique as it has been described over a century ago by Flint in 1913 as reported by Codman in 1934. After all of the various needling techniques the patient should be instructed to rest the shoulder for a short period (1 to 2 days) followed by gradual return to daily activities.

The patient should also be forewarned that a successful full recovery may take 3 to 6 mo. During the chronic formative stage the symptoms are usually mild and no intervention is needed. Yet some authors suggested needling (whether blind needling or under radiological guidance) suggesting that direct puncture of the deposits would shorten the natural history of the condition and accelerate deposits resorption. Nonsteroidal drugs may be used every now and then. The true debate concerning needling or puncture and lavage is the fact that the acute and severe symptoms are almost always associated with an expedient resolution of the condition. Thus, any form of treatment at this point will ultimately be a "success".

Operative intervention
Indications:

Many authors suggested that the indications for operative intervention include progression of symptoms that interferes with the daily activities after failure of conservative measures. Neer stated that operative indications include long standing symptoms after failure of conservative measures in the presence of multiple, hard and gritty deposits. He rarely resorted to operative intervention and suggested that residual tendinopathy would follow.

Most authors starting from Burkhead, passing through Lippmann, to Mclaughlin, and up till today agree that surgical removal of rotator cuff calcium deposits end with good permanent results. They agree that the indications include symptomatic patients after failure of conservative measures with radiological evidence of relatively homogenous calcium deposits. During the resorptive stage, conservative measures were recommended as the natural history of the condition would end with complete resolution of the deposits and the symptoms. Yet operative intervention is to be considered upon the patient's demand due to the intolerable pain despite the conservative measures.

Open surgery:

It is performed through a deltoid splitting incision, the site of which may be modified to allow the best access to the exact location of the deposits. The deltoid fibers are separated and the deposits are splitopen along the direction of the cuff fibers. Usually the deposits are readily apparent as a bulge within the cuff. The deposits commonly burst out when opened. Open surgery has a high success rate in complete removal of the calcium deposits but with some intraoperative complications.

Some authors suggested resuturing of the cuff if a significant gap is left behind. The benefit of this step is unclear. This is followed by a period of shoulder rest (5 to 7 days), with gradual return to daily activities over a 4 to 6 wk period of time.

Most authors reported that complete intraoperative removal of the deposits was unnecessary as it didn't significantly affect the final clinical outcome. Thus total removal was not essential and sometimes not possible without substantial damage to the tendon. In most cases partial removal of the deposits will finally lead to total resorption. This was reinforced by other studies.

Arthroscopic management:

Nowadays, open surgery is rarely used to remove calcium deposits as arthroscopy offers a much better choice. Arthroscopic calcium deposits removal was quite effective, although it may fail to completely remove the deposits compared with open surgery. But as long as complete removal of the deposits was unnecessary, then arthroscopic removal was clearly a better option. Studies showed that the rate of full-thickness rotator cuff tears after calcium deposits removal was quite low (3.9% after a 9-year follow-up). Accordingly, rotator cuff repair following calcium deposits removal was not mandatory. However, it was found that the intraoperative status of the rotator cuff had a significant influence on the functional results at follow-up.

In one study, the 2 patients of the 54 cases of the study (3.7%) who needed later rotator cuff repair showed obvious degeneration of the rotator cuff during the removal of the deposits. Accordingly, it should be recommended to repair the rotator cuff after the removal of calcium deposits, whenever the cuff appears to be noticeably degenerative.

Arthroscopic subacromial bursectomy should be performed to allow better visualization of the rotator cuff. In cases with shoulder impingement, subacromial decompression (acromioplasty) should be performed. The calcium deposits were identified as a bulge within the cuff tendon "calcific bulging sign". Then, *via* a lateral working portal, a half-moon arthroscopy knife may be used to open up the deposits along the fibers of the cuff. After that, a 3.5-mm motorized shaver was used to remove as much as possible of each deposit, only stopping short of causing any iatrogenic damage to the cuff.

CHAPTER EIGHT

PHYSIOTHERAPY IN CUBITAL TUNNEL SYNDROME

INTRODUCTION

Cubital tunnel syndrome occurs when the ulnar nerve or funny bone nerve is stretched, compressed, or irritated where it crosses the elbow. Exercises can help, but not all medical professionals agree on what exercises improve symptoms.

Symptoms of cubital tunnel syndrome include: numbness or tingling in the fingers, especially the ring and pinky fingers pain or soreness along the forearm weakness or soreness in the hand. The ulnar nerve extends from the neck down the back of the arm to the hand. In the inner aspect of the elbow, it runs along a small passageway called the cubital tunnel. Cubital tunnel syndrome occurs at the elbow and is also known as ulnar neuropathy.

EXERCISES

Some health experts believe certain exercises that encourage the ulnar nerve to glide gently through the cubital and Guyon's canals may improve symptoms. The cubital canal is the small channel that the ulnar nerve runs through along the inside of the elbow. Guyon's canal is where the ulnar nerve runs into the hand through the wrist.

Examples of nerve gliding exercises include:

Exercise 1

1. Extend the arm straight out in front of the body with a straightened elbow, as much as is comfortable, with the palm facing up.

2. Slowly and gently curl the fingers towards the palms then slowly and gently bend them down, away from the body.

3. Slowly and gently bend the elbow, as much as is comfortable, and then slowly release back.

Exercise 2

1. Extend the arm straight out in front of the body with a straightened elbow, as much as is comfortable, with the palm facing up.

2. Slowly and gently begin to bend the elbow towards the body while at the same time gently twisting the wrist backward, away from the body.

3. If steps 1 and 2 are comfortable, then keeping the wrist bent back, slowly and gently bends the elbow, as much as is comfortable, then slowly release it.

Exercise 3

1. Stand, sit, or lie down and extend the arm out straight alongside the body with a slightly clenched fist.

2. Slowly and gently bend the elbow, bringing the fist towards the body, as far as comfortable, and then slowly release.

Exercise 4

1. Stand with the elbow bent so that the forearm runs parallel to the body.

2. Slowly and gently twist the palms upwards to face the ceiling and then downwards to face the floor.

People should never hold the positions in cubital tunnel syndrome stretches or exercises. However, they can repeat nerve gliding and range of movement exercises for cubital tunnel syndrome 2 to 5 times each a few times each day. Doctors can sometimes recommend some range of movement exercises for people recovering from cubital tunnel syndrome surgery.

SYMPTOMS

The ulnar nerve is also sometimes called the funny bone nerve. Where the ulnar nerve crosses the elbow, there is very little fat and subcutaneous tissue, meaning the nerve is closer to the surface of the skin and more sensitive. Hence, if a person hits their inner elbow, the ensation can resemble an electric shock.

Most people with cubital tunnel syndrome experience symptoms that may include: numbness, pain, and weakness in the arm, forearm, and fingers weakened or reduced grip waking at night from pain or numbness in the hands or fingers, especially the pinky and ring fingers difficulty bending and straightening the fingers difficulty manipulating things with the hands or fingers muscle loss at the base of the small fingers. The symptoms of cubital tunnel syndrome usually get much worse when the elbow is bent for a long time or compressed.

HOME EXERCISES

Several at-home treatments may provide some relief from the symptoms of cubital tunnel syndrome. Initially, the easiest way to get relief from cubital tunnel syndrome is to avoid actions that irritate the symptoms, such as: sleeping with the elbow bent holding a phone for a long time typing for extended periods holding a book or tablet up for a long time sitting with the arms on an armrest for a long while leaning on the elbow driving for a long time driving with the arm resting on an open window.

Additional home treatment to try can include the following:

Rest the arm and elbow when possible. Apply ice compresses wrapped in a cloth or towel to the area for 10 to 15 minutes several times daily. Loosely wrap the impacted forearm with padding, such as a cloth, towel, or pillow, or wear an elbow split at night to prevent the elbow from bending. Adjust computer or writing workspaces so that the chair is not lower than the tabletop. Wear an elbow pad during the day to give protection. Avoid clothing or sports equipment that compresses or restricts the elbow. For most cases of cubital tunnel syndrome, a doctor will prescribe a splint or padded elbow brace for people to wear at night.

BRACING

Rigid nighttime bracing of the arm to keep it in a fixed position, together with moderating activity patterns, has been shown to help cubital tunnel syndrome. A 2014 study found that wearing a rigid elbow brace at night for 3 months, and avoiding activities that could irritate the ulnar nerve during the day, resolved symptoms in 21 of the 24 cases included in the study.

SURGERY

People whose symptoms are severe or last longer than 6 weeks should consult their doctor. If symptoms are extreme, chronic, or do not respond to other forms of treatment, then surgery may be necessary. Doctors may recommend surgery for people experiencing muscle loss or weakness in their hands because of cubital tunnel syndrome. In severe cases, people may continue to experience symptoms even after surgery. However, about 85 percent of people with severe nerve compression who do not respond well to other treatment options may benefit from cubital tunnel surgery.

Cubital tunnel syndrome occurs when there is pressure or strain on the ulnar nerve, also known as the funny bone nerve. Symptoms often include numbness, soreness, and weakness. Treatment may be possible with home remedies and OTC medication, or surgery may be necessary. People with symptoms of cubital tunnel syndrome should consult their doctor if they persist for more than a few weeks.

CHAPTER NINE

PHYSIOTHERAPY IN FROZEN SHOULDER

INTRODUCTION

Frozen shoulder, also known as adhesive capsulitis, is defined as *"a condition of uncertain aetiology, characterised by significant restriction of both active and passive shoulder motion that occurs in the absence of a known intrinsic shoulder disorder"*.

Patients with frozen shoulder typically experience insidious shoulder stiffness, severe pain that usually worsens at night, and near-complete loss of passive and active external rotation of the shoulder.

There are typically no significant findings in the patient's history, clinical examination or radiographic evaluation to explain the loss of motion or pain.

Frozen shoulder can be classified as primary or secondary. Primary idiopathic frozen shoulder is often associated with other diseases and conditions, such as diabetes mellitus, and may be the first presentation of a diabetic patient.

Patients with systemic diseases such as thyroid diseases and Parkinson's disease are at higher risk. Secondary adhesive capsulitis can occur after shoulder injuries or immobilisation (e.g. rotator cuff tendon tear, subacromial impingement, biceps tenosynovitis and calcific tendonitis). These patients develop pain from the shoulder pathology, leading to reduced movement in that shoulder and thus developing frozen shoulder.

Frozen shoulder often progresses in three stages: the freezing (painful), frozen (adhesive) and thawing phases. In the freezing stage, which lasts about 2–9 months, there is a gradual onset of diffuse, severe shoulder pain that typically worsens at night. The pain will begin to subside during the frozen stage with a characteristic progressive loss of glenohumeral flexion, abduction, internal rotation and external rotation. This stage can last for 4–12 months. During the thawing stage, the patient experiences a gradual return of range of motion that takes about 5–26 months to complete. Although adhesive capsulitis is often self-limiting, usually resolving in 1–3 years, it can persist, presenting symptoms that are commonly mild; pain is the most common complaint.

ROLE OF PHYSIOTHERAPIST

Most frozen shoulder cases can be managed in the primary care setting. Clinicians are encouraged to start the treatment with patient education. Explaining the natural history of the condition often helps to reduce frustration, increase compliance and allay fears for the patient. It is also advisable to acknowledge that full range of motion may never be restored. Common conservative treatments for frozen shoulder include nonsteroidal anti-inflammatory drugs (NSAIDs), glucocorticoids given orally or as intra-articular injections, and/or physical therapy. Many practitioners, however, find themselves limited to prescribing medications to relieve pain and inflammation.

Many physical therapy and home exercises can be used as a first-line treatment for adhesive capsulitis. Physical therapy has been shown to bring about pain relief and return of functional motion. When used in combination with physical therapy, NSAIDs were proven to be more effective as compared to using NSAIDs alone. Similarly, various studies on intra-articular corticosteroids used in combination with physiotherapy resulted in better outcomes compared to intra-articular corticosteroids alone.

The physical therapy for primary idiopathic frozen shoulder described herein can be useful for prescribing home exercises to increase shoulder mobility. Nevertheless, it is imperative to consider the patient's symptoms and stage of the condition when selecting a physical treatment method for frozen shoulder.

PHASES OF FROZEN SHOULDER

Freezing phase

Pain is often most severe during the freezing phase and patients in this phase would benefit from learning pain-relieving techniques. These exercises include gentle shoulder mobilisation exercises within the tolerated range (e.g. pendulum exercise, passive supine forward elevation, passive external rotation, and active assisted range of motion in extension, horizontal adduction, and internal rotation). A heat or ice pack can be applied as a modality to relieve pain before the start of these exercises. The application of moist heat in conjunction with stretching has been shown to improve muscle extensibility. Certain patients might also find it useful to take analgesics before physical therapy.

Patients should begin with short-duration (1–5 seconds) range of motion exercises, which should be in a relatively pain-free range. Pendulum exercises can be used in flexion or abduction or circular motion. Patients can also try pulley exercises, as tolerated, and neck or scapular muscle releases. It is important not to aggravate a frozen shoulder, as aggressive stretching beyond the pain threshold can result in inferior outcomes, particularly in the early phase of the condition. There has also been evidence that patients should avoid a forward shoulder posture as it may cause a loss of glenohumeral flexion and abduction.

Frozen phase

Similar to the freezing phase, a heat or ice pack can be applied during the frozen phase to relieve pain before commencing exercises. In particular, stretching exercises for the chest muscles and muscles at the back of the shoulder should be maintained. Rotation before elevation exercises, such as an external rotation stretch, is also recommended to avoid increasing pain and inflammation. At this stage, strengthening exercises are added to maintain muscle strength. Isometric or static contractions are exercises that require no joint movement and can be done without worrying about increasing pain in the shoulder.

Strengthening exercises can be performed at home. The scapular retraction exercises gently stretch the chest muscles and serve as basic strengthening for the scapular muscles. Isometric shoulder external rotation can also be used for flexion or abduction, within the available range, but care should still be taken to avoid introducing aggressive exercises, as overenthusiastic treatment could aggravate the capsular synovitis and subsequently cause pain.

Thawing phase

In the thawing phase, the patient experiences a gradual return of range of motion. It is crucial to get the shoulder back to normal as quickly as possible by regaining full movement and strength. Strengthening exercises are important, as the shoulder is considerably weakened after a few months of little movement. Compared to the frozen phase, the patient can perform more mobility exercises and stretches with a longer holding duration, within tolerated boundaries. Strengthening exercises can also progress from isometric or static contractions, to exercises using a resistance band, and eventually to free weights or weight machines. Rotator cuff exercises, as well as posture exercises and exercises for the deltoid and chest muscles, can be included in the treatment as well.

DECISION MAKING FOR REFERRAL

Referral to a physiotherapist can be made when the physician thinks that the patient's condition needs more guidance and can benefit from a physiotherapist review, or when the patient's condition fails to improve after trialling exercises such as the above. Referral to an orthopaedic specialist may be necessary if some investigations are needed, such as radiography of the shoulder (to look for calcific tendonitis or acromial bone spur, i.e. a Type 3 Bigliani spur) and magnetic resonance imaging of the shoulder to rule out cuff tear.

Manipulation of the frozen shoulder under regional anaesthesia together with intra-articular glenohumeral joint cortisone injection is an effective form of treatment in frozen shoulder without cuff tear. This is especially so if the patient would like a rapid improvement in symptoms and avoid the expected natural history of pain, stiffness and slow gradual thawing of the stiff shoulder.

CONCLUSION

- Patients with frozen shoulder typically experience insidious shoulder stiffness and near-complete loss of passive and active external rotation of the shoulder.
- Frozen shoulder occurs in three phases: freezing (painful), frozen (adhesive) and thawing, and is often self-limiting.
- Common conservative treatments for frozen shoulder include NSAIDs, glucocorticoids given orally or as intra-articular injections, and/or physical therapy.
- Physical therapy and home exercises can be a first-line treatment for frozen shoulder, with consideration of the patient's symptoms and stage of the condition.
- In the freezing (painful) stage, gentle stretching exercises can be done but should be kept within a short duration (1–5 seconds) and not go beyond the patient's pain threshold.
- In the frozen (adhesive) stage, strengthening exercises such as scapular retraction, posterior capsule stretch and isometric shoulder external rotation can be added to the patient's exercises for maintenance of

muscle strength.
- In the thawing stage, the patient experiences a gradual return of range of motion; both stretching and strengthening exercises can increase in intensity, with a longer holding duration.

CHAPTER TEN

FOCAL TASK SPECIFIC DYSTONIA

INTRODUCTION

Dystonias are a diverse "group of movement disorders characterized by sustained or intermittent muscle contractions causing abnormal, often repetitive, movements, postures, or both". Recently updated consensus opinion classifies dystonias by two axes: clinical characteristics and etiology. The first axis, clinical characteristics, includes the age of onset, affected body region, temporal pattern, and associated neurologic or systemic features. A sub-classification includes focal task specific dystonias (FTSD), which are a diverse group of focal dystonias affecting an isolated body part and are triggered, at least initially, by a specific action. While the term "dystonia" was first used in 1911 by Oppenheim, the clinical phenomenon had been described almost a century earlier in patients with FTSD. In 1830, clerks in the British Civil Service were noted to develop difficulty with writing. After observing these clerks, Sir Charles Bell remarked that he "found the action necessary for writing gone, or the motions so irregular as to make the letters be written zig-zag, whilst the power of strongly moving the arm for fencing remained". Later in the 1860s, Samuel Solly labelled this condition "scrivener's palsy". While "scrivener's palsy" or writer's cramp, as it is now called, is one of the more recognized forms of FTSD, dystonia may affect musicians, typists, hairdressers, painters, shoemakers and tailors. Sport-related FTSD have also been described in golfers, pistol shooters and ping-pong players, among others. Because of their association with repetitive, fine motor tasks often linked to one's profession, FTSD have also been referred to as occupational dystonias. Interestingly, until the 1980s FTSD were erroneously interpreted to be psychogenic in origin, often termed "occupational neuroses." In 1982, evidence for an organic etiology emerged from the work of Sheehy and Marsden.

HISTORY

FTSD typically begins in adulthood with symptom onset in the third to sixth decade. Unlike other adult onset primary focal dystonias, FTSD is more common in men, and it usually affects the arm, facial muscles or larynx. Overall prevalence estimates for FTSD in the general population range from 7 to 69 per million. However, prevalence has been estimated to be much higher in selected groups; for instance, some studies have shown as many as 14% of patients seen at performing arts medical centers have FTSD. FTSD typically presents as an insidious, painless loss of dexterity triggered by performance of a specific, often over-practiced task. Symptoms progress over time to trigger uncontrolled activation of muscle groups, leading to abnormal postures and movements. Early in the disease course, the dystonia typically is triggered only by the performance of a specific task, but over time spreads to involve other tasks, or even spreads to previously unaffected areas of the body. As with other types of dystonias, sensory tricks, or geste antagonistes, may temporarily reduce the dystonic symptoms of FTSD. Writer's cramp and musician's dystonia Writer's cramp is characterized by involuntary cramping of muscles of the hand, forearm, or upper arm selectively triggered by writing. Typically, the distal muscles of the upper extremity are affected, but dystonia may progress to include more proximal muscle groups, may be triggered by other activities, and can even spread to the opposite nondominant hand. Average age of onset is in the fourth decade, and once present, symptoms rarely remit. FTSD seen in musicians, a group that may be at risk due to overly practiced fine motor tasks, typically manifests in two phenotypes based on the particular instrument: musician's hand dystonia or embouchure dystonia. Musician's dystonia can occur in both amateur and professional musicians, men are affected four times as often as women, and average symptom onset is in the fourth decade. Musician's hand dystonia has been reported with a variety of instruments, including piano, violin, guitar, flute, clarinet, horn and tabla, among others. Dystonia typically occurs in the hand that performs the more demanding tasks, such as the right hand in pianists and the left hand in violinists. The specific pattern of abnormal muscle activation varies by instrument. For example, abnormal flexion of the fingers is typically seen in pianists and violinists, while in woodwind or brass players, extension due to lumbrical activation can occur. FTSD may be exquisitely task specific, triggered by playing one instrument, but sparing the hand when a patient plays a different instrument. Embouchure dystonia may affect brass and woodwind players, with age of onset in the fourth decade. The embouchure is the critical interplay of the lips and facial muscles with the instrument's mouthpiece that controls the production of the desired air stream. Embouchure dystonias may be further classified by the pattern of abnormal movements, including embouchure tremor, involuntary lip movements and jaw closure. In recent years, much effort has focused on understanding the etiology, risk factors and pathophysiology of FTSD and potential therapeutic interventions. We will review these in turn.

ETIOLOGY

The etiology of FTSD remains unknown, although recent lines of evidence suggest that both genetic and environmental factors are important. Examination of family members of patients with FTSD revealed up to 25% of patients with an affected family member. This is consistent with a recent study of musician's dystonia which found approximately 20% of patients with a similarly affected family member. A recent genome-wide analysis has found an association with the arylsulfatase G (ARSG) gene in both musician's hand dystonia and writer's cramp, but to date, a specific causative mutation within this gene has not been identified. Additionally, in a study of musicians with FTSD of the hand, along with patients with writer's cramp and their relatives, reduced interhemispheric inhibition as measured by transcranial magnetic stimulation (TMS) was observed in individuals where there was a positive family history for dystonia. This finding suggests that reduced interhemispheric inhibition may serve as a possible endophenotypic marker of genetic susceptibility for developing FTSD.

In addition to repetitive, over-practicing of a motor task, other environmental factors may contribute to the risk factors of developing FTSD. Possible risk factors include personality traits, such as perfectionism and anxiety, anatomical factors, such as hand size and joint mobility, as well as delayed onset of age of musical training.

PATHOPHYSIOLOGY

The pathophysiology of FTSD has been linked to abnormalities in inhibition, plasticity, and motor networks. In 1995, experiments first demonstrated decreased short intracortical inhibition (SICI) in FTSD patients compared to healthy controls using TMS. Interestingly, this abnormality was found in the bilateral hemispheres of patients, despite unilateral symptoms. Recent research has therefore postulated that decreased SICI may not directly cause abnormal motor activation but rather facilitate the development of FTSD through other mechanisms. Specifically, one suggested mechanism, found in several studies of FTSD patients, is the development of impaired surround inhibition, a neural inhibitory mechanism responsible for the selective recruitment and activation of muscles necessary for a particular task with inactivation of the neighboring muscles that are unnecessary. Consistent with the hypothesis of decreased SICI and impaired surround inhibition, multiple studies have shown a loss of dexterity and impaired independent movement of fingers of patients with either writer's cramp or musician's dystonia.

Another interesting abnormality that may contribute to FTSD pathology is maladaptive neural plasticity. While plasticity is believed to be critical to the processes of learning and memory, maladaptive neuroplastic responses in both the motor and sensory cortices have been examined in conditioning protocols using repetitive stimuli from TMS. Patients with writer's cramp exhibited abnormal responses to paired associative stimulation of the median nerve and primary motor cortex. Such abnormalities included increased facilitation with spread to non-median nerve innervated muscles in addition to the absence of a typical cortical silent period. More recently, experiments demonstrated a decreased short latency afferent inhibition following 1-Hz repetitive TMS in writer's cramp, but not in normal controls. Furthermore, in both musician's dystonia and writer's cramp, functional neuroimaging experiments have demonstrated abnormal cortical representations of digits and reorganization of the sensory homunculus in the sensory cortex. Such aberrant somatotopy may be reversible with associated improved fine motor control using constraint-induced therapy. However, another study of somatotopic mapping discovered bilateral misrepresentation of digits despite unilateral dystonic symptoms, suggesting that the disturbed somatotopy is an endophenotype for vulnerability to develop FTSD. Regardless of the etiology of the aberrant somatotopy, the evidence suggests that maladaptive plasticity of FTSD impairs sensorimotor integration.

Finally, results from recent investigations have suggested network disorder leading to FTSD, whereby involvement of the entire sensorimotor network contributes to dystonia. Hyperactivation of the basal ganglia has been demonstrated in MRI studies of writer's cramp. Further aberrant basal ganglia function has been demonstrated by PET studies, which have shown decreased release of striatal dopamine during hand activation in patients with writer's cramp. Cerebellar dysfunction has also been suggested to contribute to FTSD, although the specific abnormality is not well understood. Some investigations have reported increased cerebellar activity in patients with writer's cramp, while others have demonstrated decreased activity in the cerebellum during hand activation in FTSD. Further research is warranted to understand the precise network abnormalities; however, evidence of aberrant connections between the basal ganglia and cerebellum leading to dystonia is supported by research demonstrating that interruption of this connection leads to improvement of the dystonic symptoms.

TREATMENT

Current treatment modalities for FTSD include oral medication, chemodenervation, surgery and physical therapy. Anticholinergic agents like trihexyphenidyl, as well as other medications, such as primidone, baclofen, and phenytoin have been tried with inconsistent responses and frequent intolerable side effects. Chemodenervation with botulinum neurotoxin (BoNT) type A has been the mainstay of treatment for FTSD. Each of the seven known BoNT serotypes (types A–G) targets a specific SNARE protein for degradation in peripheral cholinergic neurons, thereby preventing the downstream release of acetylcholine into the neuromuscular junction. As a result, chemodenervation and subsequent muscle paralysis occur and persist for several months until the eventual degradation of BoNT and regeneration of SNARE proteins. While the inhibition of acetylcholine release at the neuromuscular junction is believed to be a major component of BoNT's mechanism of action, there increasing evidence that BoNT also acts peripherally at gamma motor neurons to reduce afferent sensory input from muscle spindles to the central nervous system and to alter sensorimotor pathways. Treatment of limb dystonia with BoNT has demonstrated transient increased intracortical inhibition on par with normal levels of inhibition as measured by transcranial magnetic stimulation. Furthermore, recent research suggests that BoNT may additionally have non-SNARE cellular targets involved in wide-ranging activities, such as cell division and apoptosis, neuritogenesis and gene expression. Of the seven BoNT serotypes, only serotype A and to a lesser extent serotype B are available for clinical use, with specific formulations of each serotype characterized by different potency, immunogenicity, preparation, compound stability and heat tolerance. Notably, BoNT type

B is only formally approved for the treatment of cervical dystonia, while BoNT type A has approved indications in the treatment of both neurologic and non-neurologic conditions. Multiple studies have demonstrated long-lasting treatment benefits of BoNT in FTSD, but there is a delicate balance between reducing dystonic symptoms without inducing concurrent residual weakness resulting in loss of motor function. Even with treatment, many affected musicians are no longer able to play professionally, due to the high level of fine motor skill required for continued professional performance. In recent years, emerging studies have investigated the role of surgery and sensorimotor retraining as therapeutic options. Thalamotomies have been performed as treatment of a variety of movement disorders since the 1950s. In what was the largest published case series of patients with writer's cramp undergoing stereotactic ventro-oral thalamotomy, eleven of twelve patients reported almost complete resolution of symptoms with sustained benefit for over one year after surgery. Based on its benefit for writer's cramp, stereotactic ventro-oral thalamotomy was demonstrated to improve medically refractory musician's dystonia with long-term benefit. More recently in 2016, treatment with noninvasive gamma knife ventro-oral thalamotomy was shown to be effective in a case of refractory musician's dystonia for a patient who was deemed too high-risk for conventional stereotactic thalamotomy. However, larger long-term follow-up studies will be necessary to evaluate the lasting efficacy of this intervention. Additionally, a small case series has investigated the role of deep brain stimulation (DBS) in the treatment of FTSD with promising results. Given the invasive nature of both thalamotomies and DBS, these procedures have primarily been reserved for medically refractory cases. Based on the idea of excessive motor excitability and aberrant sensorimotor integration in the development of FTSD, sensorimotor retraining may hold promise. Previous attempts at reducing focal dystonia symptoms by means of rehabilitation involved immobilization and splinting of the affected body part. Recent studies examining the effects of augmenting current rehabilitation techniques to include transcranial direct current stimulation have offered encouraging results. In 2014, patients with musician's dystonia displayed improvement of fine motor movements following motor retraining assisted by bi-hemispheric, noninvasive brain stimulation via transcranial direct current stimulation to the motor cortex. Likewise, in 2015, transcranial direct simulation was shown to enhance the response to rehabilitation in patients with FTSD of the hand in a randomized control trial. Anodal transcranial direct current stimulation targeting the cerebellum has also been shown to improve handwriting in patients with writer's cramp.

CONCLUSION

FTSD are a fascinating group of movement disorders characterized by aberrant motor overactivation during the performance of a specific, often over-practiced activity. The triggering activity can be associated with one's occupation, leading to the disorder's further classification as an occupational dystonia. The development of such a condition can impact one's livelihood, particularly if symptoms are severe. While progress has been made in recent years in understanding the etiology, risk factors and pathophysiology of FTSD, improved therapeutic options are needed.

CHAPTER ELEVEN

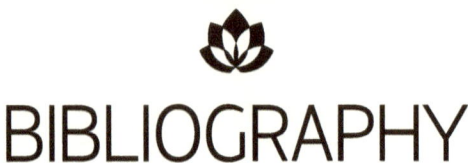

BIBLIOGRAPHY

1. Sanders TL, Maradit Kremers H, Bryan AJ, Ransom JE, Smith J, Morrey BF, et al. "The Epidemiology and Health Care Burden of Tennis Elbow: A Population-Based Study. Am J Sports Med. 2015; 43; 1066-1071.
2. Vaquero-Picado, Alfonso, Raul Barco, and Samuel A. Antuña. Lateral epicondylitis of the elbow. Effort open Rev. 2016; 11: 391-397.
3. Abrams GD, Renstrom PA, Safran MR. Epidemiology of musculoskeletal injury in the tennis player. Br J Sports Med. 2012; 46: 492-498.
4. Bylak, Joseph, and Mark R. Hutchinson. "Common sports injuries in young tennis players. Sports Med. 1998; 26: 119-132.
5. Eygendaal, Denise, F. Th G. Rahussen, and R. L. Diercks. Biomechanics of the elbow joint in tennis players and relation to pathology. *British journal of sports medicine.* 2007; 11: 820-823.
6. Kaminsky, Sean B., and Champ L. Baker. "Lateral epicondylitis of the elbow." Sports Medicine and Arthroscopy Review. 2003; 11: 63-70.
7. Rajeev A, Pooley J. Lateral compartment cartilage changes and lateral elbow pain. Acta Orthop Belg. 2009; 75: 37-40.
8. Dones VC 3rd, Grimmer K, Thoirs K, Suarez CG, Luker J. The diagnostic validity of musculoskeletal ultrasound in lateral epicondylalgia: a systematic review. BMC Med Imaging. 2014; 14: 10.
9. Cook CE, Hegedus EJ. Orthopedic Physical Examination Tests: An Evidence-Based Approach. 2016.
10. Miller TT, Shapiro MA, Schultz E, Kalish PE. Comparison of sonography and MRI for diagnosing epicondylitis. J Clin Ultrasound. 2001; 30: 193–202.
11. Tosti, Rick, John Jennings, and J. Milo Sewards. Lateral epicondylitis of the elbow. The American journal of medicine . 2013; 14: 357.

12. Bisset L, Aatit Paungmali B. Vicenzino, Elaine B. A systematic review and meta-analysis of clinical trials on physical interventions for lateral epicondylalgia. British journal of sports medicine. 2005; 39: 411-422.
13. Jafarian FS, Demneh ES, Tyson SF. The immediate effect of orthotic management on grip strength of patients with lateral epicondylosis. J Orthop Sports Phys Ther. 2009; 39: 484-499.
14. Mishra A, Pavelko T. Treatment of chronic elbow tendinosis with buffered platelet-rich plasma. Am J Sports Med. 2006; 34: 1774-1778.
15. Thanasas C, Papadimitriou G, Charalambidis C, Paraskevopoulos I, Papanikolaou A. Platelet-rich plasma versus autologous whole blood for the treatment of chronic lateral elbow epicondylitis: a randomized controlled clinical trial. Am J Sports Med. 2011 ; 39: 2130-2134.
16. Coombes BK, Bisset L, Brooks P, Khan A, Vicenzino B. Effect of corticosteroid injection, physiotherapy, or both on clinical outcomes in patients with unilateral lateral epicondylalgia: a randomized controlled trial. JAMA. 2013; 309; 461-469.
17. Lin CL, Lee JS, Su WR, Kuo LC, Tai TW, Jou IM. Clinical and ultrasonographic results of ultrasonographically guided percutaneous radiofrequency lesioning in the treatment of recalcitrant lateral epicondylitis. Am J Sports Med. 2011; 39: 2429-2435.
18. Buchbinder R, Green SE, Youd JM, Assendelft WJ, Barnsley L, Smidt N.Systematic review of the efficacy and safety of shock wave therapy for lateral elbow pain. J Rheumatol. 2006; 33: 1351-1363.
19. Gunn CC. Tennis elbow. The surgical treatment of lateral epicondylitis. JBJS .1980; 2: 313-314.
20. Rose NE, Forman SK, Dellon AL.Denervation of the lateral humeral epicondyle for treatment of chronic lateral epicondylitis. J Hand Surg Am. 2013; 38: 344-349.
21. Dunn JH, Kim JJ, Davis L, Nirschl RP. Ten-to 14-year follow-up of the Nirschl surgical technique for lateral epicondylitis. Am J Sports Med. 2008; 36: 261-266.
22. Nazar M, Lipscombe S, Morapudi S, Tuvo G, Kebrle R, Marlow W. Percutaneous tennis elbow release under local anaesthesia. Open Orthop J. 2012; 6: 129-132.
23. Pierce TP, Issa K, Gilbert BT, Hanly B1, Festa A, McInerney VK, et al. A Systematic Review of Tennis Elbow Surgery: Open Versus Arthroscopic Versus Percutaneous Release of the Common Extensor Origin. Arthroscopy. 2017; 33: 1260-1268.

24. Hoogvliet P, Randsdorp MS, Dingemanse R, Koes BW, Huisstede BM. Does effectiveness of exercise therapy and mobilisation techniques offer guidance for the treatment of lateral and medial epicondylitis? A systematic review.Br J Sports Med. 2013; 47: 1112-1119.
25. Savnik A, Jensen B, Nørregaard J, Egund N, Danneskiold-Samsøe B, Bliddal H. Magnetic resonance imaging in the evaluation of treatment response of lateral epicondylitis of the elbow. Eur Radiol. 2004; 14: 964-969.
26. Szabo SJ, Savoie FH, Field LD, Ramsey JR, Hosemann CD. Tendinosis of the extensor carpi radialis brevis: an evaluation of three methods of operative treatment. J Shoulder Elbow Surg. 2006; 15: 721-727.
27. Garcia-Porrua C, Gonza´lez-Gay MA, Ibañez D and Garcı´a-Paı´s MJ. The clinical spectrum of severe septic bursitis in north western Spain: a 10 year study. J Rheumatol 1999; 26: 663–667.
28. Perez C, Huttner A, Assal M, et al. Infectious olecranon and patellar bursitis: short-course adjuvant antibiotic therapy is not a risk factor for recurrence in adult hospitalized patients. Antimicrob Chemother 2010; 65: 1008–1014.
29. Reilly J and Nicholas JA. The chronically inflamed bursa. Clin Sport Med 1987; 6: 345–370.
30. Roschmann RA and Bell CL. Septic bursitis in immunocompromised patients. Am J Med 1987; 83: 661–665.
31. Ho G Jr and Su EY. Antibiotic therapy of septic bursitis. Its implication in the treatment of septic arthritis. Arthritis Rheum 1981; 24: 905–911.
32. Stell IM. Septic and non-septic olecranon bursitis in the accident and emergency department – an approach to management. J Accid Emerg Med 1996; 13: 351–353.
33. Ho G and Tice AD. Comparison of nonseptic and septic bursitis. Further observations on the treatment of septic bursitis. Arch Intern Med 1979; 139: 1269–1273.
34. Weinstein PS, Canoso JJ and Wohlgethan JR. Long-term follow-up of corticosteroid injection for traumatic olecranon bursitis. Ann Rheum Dis 1984; 43: 44–46.
35. Raddatz DA, Hoffman GS and Franck WA. Septic bursitis: presentation, treatment and prognosis. J Rheumatol 1987; 14: 1160–1163.
36. Shell D, Perkins R and Cosgarea A. Septic olecranon bursitis: recognition and treatment. J Am Board Fam Pract 1995; 8: 217–220.

37. Hassell AB, Fowler PD and Dawes PT. Intra-bursal tetracycline in the treatment of olecranon bursitis in patients with rheumatoid arthritis. Br J Rheumatol 1994; 33: 859–860.
38. Quayle JB and Robinson MP. A useful procedure in the treatment of chronic olecranon bursitis. Injury 1978; 9: 299–302.
39. Canoso JJ and Sheckman PR. Septic subcutaneous bursitis. Report of sixteen cases. J Rheumatol 1979; 6: 96–102.
40. Floemer F, Morrison WB, Bongartz G and Ledermann HP. MRI characteristics of olecranon bursitis. AJR Am J Roentgenol 2004; 183: 29–34.
41. Degreef I and De Smet L. Complications following resection of the olecranon bursa. Acta Orthopaedica Belgica 2006; 72: 400–403.
42. Aaron DL, Patel A, Kayiaros S and Calfee R. Four common types of bursitis: diagnosis and management. J Am Acad Orthop Surg 2011; 19: 359–367.
43. Smith DL, McAfee JH, Lucas LM, Kumar KL and Romney DM. Treatment of nonseptic olecranon bursitis. A controlled, blinded prospective trial. Arch Intern Med 1989; 149: 2527–2530.
44. So¨derquist B and Hedstro¨m SA. Predisposing factors, bacteriology and antibiotic therapy in 35 cases of septic bursitis. Scand J Infect Dis 1986; 18: 305–311.
45. Quayle JB and Robinson MP. A useful procedure in the treatment of chronic olecranon bursitis. Injury 1978; 9: 299–302.
46. Canoso JJ. Idiopathic or traumatic olecranon bursitis. Clinical features and bursal fluid analysis. Arthritis Rheum 1977; 20: 1213–1216.
47. Laupland KB and Davies HD. Olecranon septic bursitis managed in an ambulatory setting. Clin Invest Med 2001; 24: 171–178.
48. Zimmermann B III, Mikolich DJ and Ho G Jr. Septic bursitis. Semin Arthritis Rheum 1995; 24: 391–410.
49. Ho G Jr, Tice AD and Kaplan SR. Septic bursitis in the prepatellar and olecranon bursae: an analysis of 25 cases. Ann Internal Med 1978; 89: 21–27.
50. Stell IM. Management of acute bursitis: outcome study of a structured approach. J R Soc Med 1999; 92: 516–521.
51. Knight JM, Thomas JC and Maurer RC. Treatment of septic olecranon and prepatellar bursitis with percutaneous placement of a suction-irrigation system. A report of 12 cases. Clin Orthop Relat Res 1986; 206: 90–93.

52. Ogilvie-Harris DJ and Gilbart M. Endoscopic bursal resection: the olecranon bursa and prepatellar bursa. Arthroscopy 2000; 16: 249–253.
53. Dillon JP, Freedman I, Tan JS, Mitchell D and English S. Endoscopic bursectomy for the treatment of septic prepatellar bursitis: a case series. Arch Orthop Trauma Surg 2012; 132: 921–925.
54. Albanese A et al (2013) Phenomenology and classification of dystonia: a consensus update. Mov Disord 28(7):863–873.
55. Oppenheim H (1911) Text-book of nervous diseases for physicians and students. 5th enl. and improved ed. O. Schulze & company, Edinburgh. G. E. Stechert & company, New York.
56. Bell C (1933) Partial paralyses of the muscles of the extremities'. The nervous system of the human body. Taylor and Francis, London, pp 57–58
57. Pearce JM (2005) A note on scrivener's palsy. J Neurol Neurosurg Psychiatry 76(4):513.
58. Frucht SJ (2004) Focal task-specific dystonia in musicians. Adv Neurol 94:225–230
59. Frucht SJ et al (2001) The natural history of embouchure dystonia. Mov Disord 16(5):899–906.
60. Yoo SW et al (2015) Hairdresser dystonia: an unusual substantia nigra hyperechogenicity. J Neurol Sci 357(1–2):314–316
61. Sheehy MP, Marsden CD (1982) Writers' cramp-a focal dystonia. Brain 105(Pt 3):461–480
62. Defazio G, Berardelli A, Hallett M (2007) Do primary adult-onset focal dystonias share aetiological factors? Brain 130(Pt 5):1183–1193
63. Epidemiological Study of Dystonia in Europe Collaborative, G (2000) A prevalence study of primary dystonia in eight European countries. J Neurol 247(10):787–792
64. Butler AG et al (2004) An epidemiologic survey of dystonia within the entire population of northeast England over the past nine years. Adv Neurol 94:95–99
65. Altenmuller E (2003) Focal dystonia: advances in brain imaging and understanding of fine motor control in musicians. Hand Clin 19(3):523–538 (xi)
66. Brandfonbrener A (1995) Musicians with focal dystonia: a report of 58 cases seen during a ten-year period at a performing arts medicine clinic. Med Probl Perform Artists 10:121–127

67. Greene PE, Bressman S (1998) Exteroceptive and interoceptive stimuli in dystonia. Mov Disord 13(3):549–551
68. Conti AM, Pullman S, Frucht SJ (2008) The hand that has forgotten its cunning—lessons from musicians' hand dystonia. Mov Disord 23(10):1398–1406
69. Altenmuller E, Jabusch HC (2010) Focal dystonia in musicians: phenomenology, pathophysiology and triggering factors. Eur J Neurol 17(Suppl 1):31–36
70. Schmidt A et al (2013) Challenges of making music: what causes musician's dystonia? JAMA Neurol 70(11):1456–1459
71. Waddy HM et al (1991) A genetic study of idiopathic focal dystonias. Ann Neurol 29(3):320–324
72. Stojanovic M, Cvetkovic D, Kostic VS (1995) A genetic study of idiopathic focal dystonias. J Neurol 242(8):508–511
73. Schmidt A et al (2009) Etiology of musician's dystonia: familial or environmental? Neurology 72(14):1248–1254
74. Lohmann K et al (2014) Genome-wide association study in musician's dystonia: a risk variant at the arylsulfatase G locus? Mov Disord 29(7):921–927
75. Nibbeling E et al (2015) Accumulation of rare variants in the arylsulfatase G (ARSG) gene in task-specific dystonia. J Neurol 262(5):1340–1343
76. Baumer T et al (2016) Abnormal interhemispheric inhibition in musician's dystonia—trait or state? Parkinsonism Relat Disord 25:33–38
77. Ioannou CI, Altenmuller E (2014) Psychological characteristics in musicians dystonia: a new diagnostic classification. Neuropsychologia 61:80–88
78. Leijnse JN, Hallett M, Sonneveld GJ (2015) A multifactorial conceptual model of peripheral neuromusculoskeletal predisposing factors in task-specific focal hand dystonia in musicians: etiologic and therapeutic implications. Biol Cybern 109(1):109–123
79. Ridding MC et al (1995) Changes in the balance between motor cortical excitation and inhibition in focal, task specific dystonia. J Neurol Neurosurg Psychiatry 59(5):493–498
80. Beck S et al (2008) Short intracortical and surround inhibition are selectively reduced during movement initiation in focal hand dystonia. J Neurosci 28(41):10363–10369

81. Hallett M (2011) Neurophysiology of dystonia: the role of inhibition. Neurobiol Dis 42(2):177–184
82. Beck S, Hallett M (2011) Surround inhibition in the motor system. Exp Brain Res 210(2):165–172
83. Sohn YH, Hallett M (2004) Disturbed surround inhibition in focal hand dystonia. Ann Neurol 56(4):595–599
84. Furuya S et al (2015) Losing dexterity: patterns of impaired coordination of finger movements in musician's dystonia. Sci Rep 5:13360
85. Furuya S, Altenmuller E (2013) Finger-specific loss of independent control of movements in musicians with focal dystonia. Neuroscience 247:152–163
86. Curra A et al (2004) Impairment of individual finger movements in patients with hand dystonia. Mov Disord 19(11):1351–1357
87. Siebner HR, Rothwell J (2003) Transcranial magnetic stimulation: new insights into representational cortical plasticity. Exp Brain Res 148(1):1–16
88. Quartarone A et al (2003) Abnormal associative plasticity of the human motor cortex in writer's cramp. Brain 126(Pt 12):2586–2596
89. Baumer T et al (2007) Abnormal plasticity of the sensorimotor cortex to slow repetitive transcranial magnetic stimulation in patients with writer's cramp. Mov Disord 22(1):81–90
90. Elbert T et al (1998) Alteration of digital representations in somatosensory cortex in focal hand dystonia. Neuroreport 9(16):3571–3575
91. Nelson AJ, Blake DT, Chen R (2009) Digit-specific aberrations in the primary somatosensory cortex in Writer's cramp. Ann Neurol 66(2):146–154
92. Bara-Jimenez W et al (1998) Abnormal somatosensory homunculus in dystonia of the hand. Ann Neurol 44(5):828–831
93. Candia V et al (2003) Effective behavioral treatment of focal hand dystonia in musicians alters somatosensory cortical organization. Proc Natl Acad Sci USA 100(13):7942–7946
94. Candia V et al (2002) Sensory motor retuning: a behavioural treatment for focal hand dystonia of pianists and guitarists. Arch Phys Med Rehabil 83(10):1342–1348
95. Candia V et al (1999) Constraint-induced movement therapy for focal hand dystonia in musicians. Lancet 353(9146):42

96. Meunier S et al (2001) Human brain mapping in dystonia reveals both endophenotypic traits and adaptive reorganization. Ann Neurol 50(4):521–527
97. Furuya S, Hanakawa T (2016) The curse of motor expertise: usedependent focal dystonia as a manifestation of maladaptive changes in body representation. Neurosci Res 104:112–119
98. Blood AJ et al (2004) Basal ganglia activity remains elevated after movement in focal hand dystonia. Ann Neurol 55(5):744–748
99. Berman BD et al (2013) Striatal dopaminergic dysfunction at rest and during task performance in writer's cramp. Brain 136(Pt 12):3645–3658
100. Odergren T, Stone-Elander S, Ingvar M (1998) Cerebral and cerebellar activation in correlation to the action-induced dystonia in writer's cramp. Mov Disord 13(3):497–508
101. Preibisch C et al (2001) Cerebral activation patterns in patients with writer's cramp: a functional magnetic resonance imaging study. J Neurol 248(1):10–17
102. Lerner A et al (2004) Regional cerebral blood flow correlates of the severity of writer's cramp symptoms. Neuroimage 21(3):904–913
103. Kadota H et al (2010) An fMRI study of musicians with focal dystonia during tapping tasks. J Neurol 257(7):1092–1098
104. Moore RD et al (2012) Individuated finger control in focal hand dystonia: an fMRI study. Neuroimage 61(4):823–831
105. Chen CH et al (2014) Short latency cerebellar modulation of the basal ganglia. Nat Neurosci 17(12):1767–1775
106. Jabusch HC et al (2005) Focal dystonia in musicians: treatment strategies and long-term outcome in 144 patients. Mov Disord 20(12):1623–1626
107. Jankovic J (2006) Treatment of dystonia. Lancet Neurol 5(10):864–872
108. Balash Y, Giladi N (2004) Efficacy of pharmacological treatment of dystonia: evidence-based review including meta-analysis of the effect of botulinum toxin and other cure options. Eur J Neurol 11(6):361–370
109. Simpson LL (2004) Identification of the major steps in botulinum toxin action. Annu Rev Pharmacol Toxicol 44:167–193
110. Rosales RL, Dressler D (2010) On muscle spindles, dystonia and botulinum toxin. Eur J Neurol 17(Suppl 1):71–80
111. Rosales RL et al (1996) Extrafusal and intrafusal muscle effects in experimental botulinum toxin-A injection. Muscle Nerve 19(4):488–496

112. Palomar FJ, Mir P (2012) Neurophysiological changes after intramuscular injection of botulinum toxin. Clin Neurophysiol 123(1):54–60
113. Matak I, Lackovic Z (2014) Botulinum toxin A, brain and pain. Prog Neurobiol 119–120:39–59
114. Giladi N (1997) The mechanism of action of botulinum toxin type A in focal dystonia is most probably through its dual effect on efferent (motor) and afferent pathways at the injected site. J Neurol Sci 152(2):132–135 Gilio F et al (2000) Effects of botulinum toxin type A on intracortical inhibition in patients with dystonia. Ann Neurol 48(1):20–26
115. Matak I, Lackovic Z (2015) Botulinum neurotoxin type A: actions beyond SNAP-25? Toxicology 335:79–84
116. Bentivoglio AR et al (2015) Clinical differences between botulinum neurotoxin type A and B. Toxicon 107(Pt A):77–84
117. Hallett M et al (2013) Evidence-based review and assessment of botulinum neurotoxin for the treatment of movement disorders. Toxicon 67:94–114
118. Lungu C et al (2011) Long-term follow-up of botulinum toxin therapy for focal hand dystonia: outcome at 10 years or more. Mov Disord 26(4):750–753
119. Mejia NI, Vuong KD, Jankovic J (2005) Long-term botulinum toxin efficacy, safety, and immunogenicity. Mov Disord 20(5):592–597
120. Schuele S et al (2005) Botulinum toxin injections in the treatment of musician's dystonia. Neurology 64(2):341–343
121. Andrew J, Fowler CJ, Harrison MJ (1983) Stereotaxic thalamotomy in 55 cases of dystonia. Brain 106(Pt 4):981–1000
122. Taira T, Hori T (2003) Stereotactic ventrooralis thalamotomy for task-specific focal hand dystonia (writer's cramp). Stereotact Funct Neurosurg 80(1–4):88–91
123. Horisawa S et al (2013) Long-term improvement of musician's dystonia after stereotactic ventro-oral thalamotomy. Ann Neurol 74(5):648–654
124. Horisawa S et al (2016) Gamma knife ventro-oral thalamotomy for musician's dystonia. Mov Disord
125. Fukaya C et al (2007) Thalamic deep brain stimulation for writer's cramp. J Neurosurg 107(5):977–982
126. Furuya S et al (2014) Surmounting retraining limits in musicians' dystonia by transcranial stimulation. Ann Neurol 75(5):700–707

127. Rosset-Llobet J, Fabregas-Molas S, Pascual-Leone A (2015) Effect of transcranial direct current stimulation on neurorehabilitation of task-specific dystonia: a double-blind, randomized clinical trial. Med Probl Perform Artists 30(3):178–184
128. Bradnam LV et al (2015) Anodal transcranial direct current stimulation to the cerebellum improves handwriting and cyclic drawing kinematics in focal hand dystonia. Front Hum Neurosci 9:286
129. Halder AM, Zhao KD, Driscoll SWO, Morrey BF, An KN. Dynamic contributions to superior shoulder stability. J Orthop Res. 2001;19(1001):206–12.
130. Randelli P, Spennacchio P, Ragone V, Arrigoni P, Casella A, Cabitza P. Complications associated with arthroscopic rotator cuff repair: a literature review. Musculoskelet Surg. 2012;96(1):9–16.
131. Huberty D, Schoolfield J, Brady P, Vadala AP, Arrigoni P, Burkhart SS. Incidence and treatment of postoperative stiffness following arthroscopic rotator cuff repair. Arthrosc J Arthrosc Relat Surg. 2009;25(8):880–90.
132. Brislin KJ, Field LD, Iii FHS. Complications after arthroscopic rotator cuff repair. Arthrosc J Arthrosc Relat Surg. 2007;23(2): 124–8.
133. Audige L, Blum R, Muller AM, Flury M, Durchholz H. Complications following arthroscopic rotator cuff tear repair: a systematic review of terms and definitions with focus on shoulder stiffness. Am J Sports Med. 3(6):2325967115587861.

www.ingramcontent.com/pod-product-compliance
Lightning Source LLC
Chambersburg PA
CBHW030849180526
45163CB00004B/1509